The Peace of Mind
PRESCRIPTION

The Peace of Mind
PRESCRIPTION

AN AUTHORITATIVE GUIDE TO FINDING
THE MOST EFFECTIVE TREATMENT
FOR ANXIETY AND DEPRESSION

DENNIS S. CHARNEY, M.D., and
CHARLES B. NEMEROFF, M.D., PH.D.
WITH STEPHEN BRAUN

HOUGHTON MIFFLIN COMPANY

BOSTON   NEW YORK   2004

For information about permission to reproduce selections from this book, write to Permissions, Houghton Mifflin Company, 215 Park Avenue South, New York, New York 10003.

Visit our Web site: www.houghtonmifflinbooks.com.

ISBN-13: 978-0-618-33502-2
ISBN-10: 0-618-33502-1

Library of Congress Cataloging-in-Publication Data

Charney, Dennis S.
The peace of mind prescription : an authoritative guide to finding the most effective treatment for anxiety and depression / Dennis S. Charney and Charles B. Nemeroff, with Stephen Braun.
p. cm.
ISBN 0-618-33502-1
1. Depression, Mental — Treatment.   2. Manic-depressive illness — Treatment.   3. Anxiety — Treatment.   4. Depression, Mental — Alternative treatment.   5. Manic-depressive illness — Alternative treatment.   6. Anxiety — Alternative treatment.   7. Peace of mind.   I. Braun, Stephen.   II. Nemeroff, Charles B.   III. Title.

RC537. C459 2004
616.85′27 — dc22   2004040530

Printed in the United States of America

QUM 10 9 8 7 6 5 4 3 2 1

To the most important people in my life: my wife, Gayle, for supporting me, loving me, and tolerating the long hours without a complaint; Gigi, Ross, Mandy, and Michael, for being the most wonderful, challenging, kind, and supportive children anyone could hope for; my sister Elaine, who has always been there for me; and my patients, colleagues, students, teachers, staff, and friends, for all they have taught me

— CHARLES B. NEMEROFF

To my wife, life partner, and best friend, Andrea; our children, Alex, Allison, Danielle, Lauren, and Meredith, who make us tremendously proud by being the people they have become, and our friend Dorinne Naughton, who is an inspiration to us all

— DENNIS S. CHARNEY

Contents

The Peace of Mind
PRESCRIPTION

EMPOWERING PEOPLE
WITH ANXIETY
AND DEPRESSION

> In the midst of winter, I finally learned that there was in me an invincible summer.
>
> — ALBERT CAMUS, *Summer*

ANXIETY AND DEPRESSION are two of the most serious medical disorders. The suffering caused by these conditions is not only miserable, grinding, and so intolerable that suicide can appear a welcome relief, but it is diabolically long-lasting if not treated. We used to view anxiety and depression as afflictions of middle age. We now know that they strike the young with equal force and can be ruinous throughout life unless treated. We used to think that anxiety and depression were purely mental ills — disorders of emotion, thinking, and perspective. In fact, anxiety and depression are deeply rooted in the body, and their corrosive effects raise a person's risk of contracting a host of diseases, including heart disease, stroke, diabetes, and osteoporosis.

Depression alone is the leading cause of disability in the United States and the rest of the world.[1] It costs employers an estimated $44 billion a year in lost productivity, according to a 2003 article in the *Journal of the American Medical Association.*[2] Tragically, not only is the true magnitude of the damage wrought by these diseases widely unknown, but millions of people do not recognize their own anxiety or depression, or if they do, they suppress this recognition because of the stigma that stubbornly clings to psychological conditions of all kinds.

This book is our attempt to fight that stigma, raise awareness about the true nature of anxiety and depression, help people find optimal treat-

1

ment, and empower them so they can better navigate often complicated health-care systems.

We live in remarkably stressful times, filled with information overload, demands to perform at high speed, and pressure to multitask. The terrorism and war that have touched all of us in recent years have also added uncertainty and tension to our lives. Unfortunately, humans are not built for this kind of stress. Our brains, our moods, and our emotional responses evolved over millions of years to deal with the challenges of a hunter-gatherer lifestyle, in which new information came at a trickle and the pace of life was, literally, at a walk. The contrast with the demands of the twenty-first century is so stark that the steady rise in anxiety and depression is not surprising. Between 1987 and 1997, for example, the percentage of Americans diagnosed and treated for depression more than tripled.[3] Anxiety and depression are now the two most common mental disorders, affecting 38 million people in the United States alone.[4]

We urgently want to address these dire statistics by improving care for those who are anxious, depressed, or both. Until now no comprehensive and authoritative guide has existed for people seeking the optimal treatment they deserve. In part, that's because until recently experts have considered anxiety and depression separate maladies. We now know this is false: people often experience symptoms of both, and proper diagnosis and treatment require an appreciation for the interrelatedness of these two disorders.

This book offers the most up-to-date and high-quality information available anywhere about the science and treatment of anxiety and depression. Our recommendations, suggestions, and guidance are grounded in evidence-based medicine, which simply means that we back up our assertions with findings from recent well-designed studies published in peer-reviewed professional journals. We have been fortunate to be involved with dozens of such studies, thousands of patients, and key national patient-advocacy groups. One of us, Dennis S. Charney, oversees scores of research projects every year as chief of Mood and Anxiety Disorder Research at the National Institute of Mental Health. The other, Charles B. Nemeroff, is a professor and chair of the Department of Psychiatry and Behavioral Sciences at Emory University, a leading center for research, training, and clinical care of patients with mood and anxiety disorders. He has treated many of the patients whose stories appear in this book. Because of our prominence in the field, we often consult with leading companies involved in treating anxiety and depression. In the spirit of full disclosure, we list these relationships in the endnotes.[5] Such arrangements, very common in psychiatry, are mutually beneficial and do not compromise our commitment to writing a book based solely on the state of the science and weight of the latest medical evidence.

Our understanding of anxiety and depression is not just a matter of long clinical experience and formal academic training, however. We are not removed from the conditions about which we write. We have our own human foibles and have experienced our share of grief, tragedy, and pain. We would never pretend to know exactly how anybody else feels, but we do have a profound empathy and compassion for everyone who struggles with anxiety and depression — an empathy rooted in our own struggles with life's slings and arrows.

Our fundamental message is hopeful: people can overcome anxiety and depression and find well-being, zest, and greater emotional resilience. Everyone can make progress. Everyone can get better. Everyone can be happier and healthier. We're not saying the path will be easy, quick, or painless, but we are certain that good information is the foundation for any successful treatment — and that is what this book contains.

In tackling anxiety or depression, recognize a fact sometimes overlooked by physicians and the medical establishment in general: nobody knows more about you than you do, and you may understand yourself better than you realize. That doesn't mean you are all-knowing or have plumbed the depths of your own multilayered consciousness. It simply means that you are the ultimate judge of when you need help, when you feel well, and when you think a change is needed in your treatment plan. Like most people, you are wiser and stronger than you may think you are. In the grip of depression or anxiety, you may minimize or dismiss your ability to change, heal, and grow, and this self-doubt is in fact part of the insidious nature of these illnesses.

Though we cannot hear your story directly or tailor what we have to offer to your particular circumstances, we acknowledge the primacy of your own unique life and all of the strengths and weaknesses you bring to bear on dealing with challenges to your health and well-being. There is no magic formula, no "absolutely effective" therapy, no "best" medication that works for everyone. You must weigh the ideas, suggestions, and options presented in this book against your own life, your own values, your own situation, and then act.

NOT JUST TREATMENT, BUT OPTIMAL TREATMENT

Sadly, millions of people with anxiety and depression are not achieving the relief they deserve. Only about one in five of those with major depression gets adequate treatment, according to a 2003 study. "Adequate" was defined as at least eight half-hour sessions of counseling with a mental health professional or four visits with any type of physician for prescription and management of an antidepressant drug, used for at least thirty days.[6]

Many people simply don't realize they are sadder, more tired, or more anxious than they need to be. Others know they suffer but don't seek treatment out of fear, embarrassment, or shame. Such concerns persist despite decades of testimony by people from all walks of life that anxiety and depression are medical conditions just like any other. Nobody is embarrassed to admit they have high blood pressure or diabetes, and nobody should be embarrassed to admit they are dealing with anxiety or depression. Almost all medical diseases involve complicated interactions between mind and body, and no clear distinction can be drawn between "physical illnesses" and "mental illnesses." Unfortunately, this relatively new way of looking at illness has not become common knowledge.

Even people currently receiving treatment often do not get optimal treatment. Their psychotherapy may be stuck or simply not working. Their medication dose may be too low, it may have lost its effectiveness, or perhaps it wasn't effective to begin with. Efforts to adopt a healthier lifestyle may be bogged down because of lack of time, money, or energy. This book offers many suggestions for overcoming barriers and getting the treatment one deserves.

It's also true that despite the breakthroughs of the past two decades, treating anxiety and depression is a complicated and still inexact science. Don't get us wrong — we have the tools, both psychotherapeutic and pharmacological, to heal most of the people who seek help. But clinicians need skill and experience in order to use these tools correctly, and patience and commitment on the part of both the patient and the clinician are essential. Often people need to try a number of approaches until one, or a combination, works. If the search continues for months, people may stop before they have wrung the most from today's arsenal of treatments. Don't accept a "quick fix" approach. A brief medical history, a fifteen-minute chat with a family doctor, and a prescription for an antidepressant or anti-anxiety medication are seldom enough. Everyone deserves more — a true therapeutic alliance with attention to the subtleties, both physical and psychological, that determine how well and rapidly a person will overcome anxiety or depression.

USING THIS BOOK

We have organized this book in three parts. Part I covers basic information relevant to everyone and is important for understanding later chapters. Part II covers the diagnosis and treatment of anxiety and depression. Part III explores how anxiety and depression affect people at different stages of life. The appendixes contain valuable information about special topics such as complementary therapies, how to evaluate health information claims, and where to find nearby psychiatric help.

The stories of real people and their struggles with anxiety and depression are woven into every part of the book. Some patients have allowed use of their real names because they want to combat the stigma lingering around anxiety and depression. Others have chosen anonymity out of concern for the privacy of others involved in their story. We are deeply grateful to all of them for sharing some of the most difficult or painful times of their lives. We believe these stories add an invaluable dimension to the factual information we present.

A few anxiety-related afflictions are not addressed in this book. For instance, we do not discuss obsessive-compulsive disorder (OCD) because current research suggests it is a distinct psychiatric entity that should not be lumped with other anxiety disorders. Although patients with OCD need as much help as any, this subject is better treated in a book of its own. Interested readers might consider *The Boy Who Couldn't Stop Washing: The Experience and Treatment of Obsessive-Compulsive Disorder,* by Judith Rapoport.[7] We also do not specifically cover so-called simple phobias — abnormal reactions to specific things such as snakes, spiders, or blood. Such phobias are relatively uncommon in the general population (as opposed to simply disliking or fearing snakes or spiders). In addition, simple phobias are seldom disabling, and their treatment is relatively straightforward.

We have written this book because we know that healing and happiness are possible, and people can lead more rewarding, satisfying, and pleasurable lives by taking advantage of everything we know about anxiety and depression. By opening this book you have already taken the immensely important step of seeking help and information. We wish you courage, patience, and tenacity as you apply what you learn here to your own life and loved ones.

PART I

The Power
of Mood

1

Thieves of Happiness

The Brain is wider than the Sky —
For — put them side by side —
The one the other will contain
With ease — and You — beside.

— Emily Dickinson

THE MALADIES TODAY called anxiety and depression can be detected in the works of ancient writers from Galen, the Greek father of medicine, to Confucius. The descriptions, however, often don't fit into the tidy diagnostic boxes used today. Take, for example, this passage from the Book of Job:

Months of Delusion I have assigned for me
Nothing for my own but nights of grief
Lying in my bed, I wonder when will it be day?
Risen I think how slowly evening comes.
Restlessly I fret till twilight falls
Swifter than a weaver's shuttle my days have passed
And vanished leaving no hope behind.

Job is clearly depressed — the hopelessness, nights of grief, and sense of meaninglessness are all there. And yet Job also seems anxious, restlessly fretting his way through the day until twilight falls.

Job's symptoms are actually very common — but recognition of the coexistence of anxiety and depression has come only recently to the medical and psychiatric professions. We now know that about half of those with an anxiety disorder also have some symptoms of depression, and, conversely, half of those who are depressed also suffer symptoms of anxiety.[1] The same types of life stressors (child abuse, trauma, conflict, and so on) raise one's vulnerability to both anxiety and depression. And medications originally developed as antidepressants are equally effective against some anxiety disorders.

9

In short, the labels *anxiety* and *depression* are often too simplistic to describe the experiences of real people. But we will use these terms, and we'll discuss anxiety and depression separately in the chapters to come, because, in day-to-day practice, enough differences exist between the two disorders and the way they are treated that a division is warranted. It pays to remember their interconnectedness, however, because it can unify both the conception and treatment of these disorders.

This chapter provides background information relevant to both disorders, which will be needed to understand later discussions. We begin with a look at why anxiety and depression exist in the first place. Why have these crippling and intensely painful diseases survived millions of years of natural selection? To explore the answer, consider the following story about one of the more bizarre conditions known to medical science.

THE STRANGE TALE OF "MISS C."

In 1928 a baby girl was born in Montreal to a physician and his wife. It was a normal delivery, and the little girl appeared healthy in every way. But as the months passed, her parents began to feel that there was something odd about the child.[2]

According to her own reports given in an interview years later, she was a "highly excitable" child who hit herself or bit her tongue and hands when frustrated. Though these behaviors troubled her parents, the child herself seemed curiously oblivious to the cuts or bruises that resulted. Then, when she was almost two years old, she developed a large, soft swelling on the back of her head — an abscess that resembled a large blister. A doctor drained the abscess at the hospital, and the procedure was utterly unremarkable except for one thing: the little girl showed no signs of pain during or after the procedure.

As the years wore on, the startling truth of the girl's condition became distressingly obvious: she could not feel pain. She never had a headache. She never had a toothache, a stomachache, an earache, or any discomfort from cuts or bruises. She also never felt an itch — even when exposed to chickenpox, sunburn, or the dry air of the long Canadian winters, which made those around her miserable with the overpowering urge to scratch.

Although at first glance an inability to feel pain sounds like a highly attractive "disorder," both the girl and her parents knew better. In fact, her extremely rare condition was life-threatening — a fact made clear one winter's day. Alone in her room, the girl heard some children playing in the snowy street outside. She went to her window and, in order to see more clearly, knelt on a scalding hot radiator. Minutes passed before she grew tired of watching the street scene. Then she got off the radiator and walked away.

Her parents discovered the burns immediately and rushed her to the hospital. There she underwent extensive skin grafts to repair the damage.

The girl was formally evaluated in 1948, and in the published account of her case she was dubbed "Miss C." to protect her privacy. By then, Miss C.'s hands, legs, and feet were scarred from cuts, bites, burns, scratches, and frostbite. In addition, her tongue had become deformed from severe biting — some intentional during childhood, some unintentional in later years as a result of normal accidents during eating, which went unnoticed. She had also been hospitalized repeatedly for serious bacterial infections of her joints.

When normal people twist an ankle, sprain a muscle, or overextend a joint, the pain caused by the tissue damage forces protective measures. Crutches are used, a muscle is favored, a joint is immobilized. Miss C., with her pain alarm system disabled, was deaf to her body's screams. She would continue to walk on a sprained ankle, use a torn muscle, or flex a damaged joint. Only when bacteria infected the area, causing it to become red and swollen, would she become aware of the problem.

Thanks to antibiotics, Miss C. survived these infections, had a relatively normal upbringing, and graduated from college. She was described in the published report as "very capable and cooperative and displaying remarkable initiative" in her work as an assistant in the psychology division of the Allan Memorial Institute.

But her health problems became worse.

Her bones and joints began to break down and become deformed from years of unintentional punishment. She could no longer walk, and the infections became more severe.

In 1957, Miss C. was hospitalized for the last time, again because of massive bacterial infections. The trauma occurring in Miss C.'s tissues finally reached such monumental proportions that she began to feel pain for the first time in her life. Traditional analgesia eased that pain, but even the most powerful antibiotics were useless. A month after she was admitted to the hospital, at the age of twenty-nine, Miss C. was dead.

THE LOGIC OF PAIN

Miss C.'s sad story is a vivid reminder that pain exists for good reasons — it promotes survival by signaling bodily damage and triggering learning so that dangerous situations can be avoided in the future. In a similar way, painful emotional states such as anxious or depressed moods exist because they serve a valuable purpose. Indeed, such feelings are vital bodily responses honed by millions of years of natural selection.[3] For instance, anxious feelings alert us to potential threats or danger. Anxiety can also motivate. The stress that builds up as one procrastinates before a deadline is unpleasant but potentially helpful.

Depressed moods can also be unpleasant but useful — especially for extremely social animals such as human beings. A depressed mood often signals that something or someone is reducing our chances for survival, reproduction, and well-being. Loss, for example, often creates a depressed mood — loss of a loved one, social status or position, security, financial means, and so on. Nature may also favor the survival of depressed moods because they provide a temporarily valuable clarity of mind.

Several studies have demonstrated that mildly depressed moods confer a uniquely keen view of the world. It appears that "normal" human beings have a somewhat rosy view of themselves and their position in life. Such a view encourages behaviors, such as seeking status or mates, that increase the chances of survival and procreation. The rosy glasses are dropped, however, in a depressed mood. People who are mildly depressed better predict their performance relative to others, better understand the limits of their control, and more accurately monitor and assess their own social behavior. The sometimes harsh reality revealed by a depressed mood — called depressive realism — may thus allow a more accurate appraisal of a situation and lead to a more successful outcome.

Notice that we have been saying "anxiety," not "anxiety disorder," and "depressed mood," not "depression." That's because occasional anxiety in the face of a real threat and occasional depressed mood in response to a real or threatened loss are normal and adaptive.

But anxiety disorders and depression are *not* normal and *not* adaptive. These serious, sometimes life-threatening illnesses confer no benefits to an individual. For example, the depressive realism characteristic of a mild depressed mood disappears in true depression and becomes unrealistic pessimism: a warped and dismal view of the world, not based on reality. Anxiety disorders and depression are dysfunctions of the elaborate systems designed by nature for our own protection and welfare, just as some forms of chronic pain are malfunctions of our elaborate pain-sensing systems.

Treating anxiety disorders and depression, therefore, does not mean obliterating one's capacity to feel anxiety or a depressed mood. Rather, the goal is eradicating dysfunction and restoring a healthy capacity for negative emotions in the same way that good pain management erases severe pain without destroying the fundamental capacity to feel pain.

Of course, anxiety and depression both range in severity from nonexistent to paralyzingly severe. When symptoms are close to the "normal" end of the spectrum, it can be tricky to decide if they warrant treatment. It's important to pay attention to anxious or depressed moods because they may be signaling trouble in one's life. For instance, job or relationship stress may be causing symptoms that should be dealt with by reducing the stress rather than adjusting the brain to accommodate the stress.

That said, the definition of "normal mood" has changed with the ready availability of safe medications for anxiety and depression. This isn't necessarily cause for alarm. Prior to the invention of eyeglasses it was "normal" for many people to have horrible eyesight. Some advances in science or technology really do improve the quality of life even when they make us less "natural." In our practices we have seen many mildly depressed people, who might have been considered "normal" fifty years ago, bloom when they have received treatment — and that treatment often involves both psychotherapy and at least short-term medication.

Most people struggling with anxiety or depression, however, are quite far from normal, and their symptoms are obviously debilitating. Making progress against these disorders requires some preliminary understanding of the organ most directly involved — the brain — and how it connects to the rest of the body.

THE BRAIN BEHIND THE MIND

The brain is a wet, wrinkled lump of squishy tissue that generates all of our memories, emotions, and self-awareness. The brain's amazing capabilities appear, on the face of it, so unlikely that for centuries thinkers looked for more plausible explanations of its workings. Aristotle believed that the brain merely radiated excess heat, and according to a nineteenth-century notion, a homunculus (little man) lived inside the brain and did its seeing, thinking, and acting.

The brain is hard to grasp, in part, because its working units — cells called neurons — are microscopic and "wired" together in astonishing complexity. Even today, when engineers can cram 100 million transistors onto a computer chip the size of a thumbnail, the brain's machinery remains impressive. The average brain contains about 100 billion neurons, but that doesn't begin to convey its true complexity and sophistication.

From the body of a typical neuron sprout thousands of branches that are linked to other neurons. Each branch, or dendrite, receives incoming messages from other neurons in the form of tiny electrochemical pulses. The messages say either "Fire" or "Don't fire." If enough "fire" messages are received, a kind of switch is flipped, and a new electrochemical impulse shoots out of the cell along a single large extension called an axon.

Signals are shuttled in this way between the brain's billions of neu-

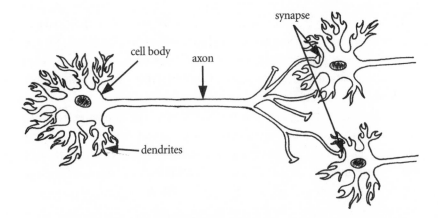

FIGURE 1A. *The main features of a typical neuron.* Dendrites communicate nerve impulses arriving from other neurons to the body of the nerve cell. If the cell receives enough stimulatory impulses, it generates an electrochemical impulse that travels down an axon. At the end of the axon the impulse triggers the release of molecules called neurotransmitters, which cross a small space — the synapse — and bind to receptors on the dendrites or cell body of another neuron. The branches of the axon may form synapses with as many as a thousand other neurons.

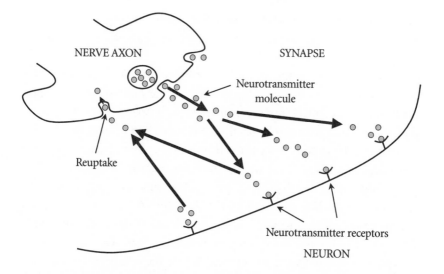

FIGURE 1B. *Neurotransmission.* Neurotransmitter molecules secreted by a nerve axon first cross the synapse and momentarily bind to receptors on the next neuron. Some neurotransmitters are then cleared from the synapse through reuptake, by the sending axon terminal.

rons. Yet the neurons don't actually touch. They are separated by tiny fluid-filled gaps called synapses. When an electrochemical signal racing down an axon gets to the end of the axon, it causes dozens of little packets of molecules called neurotransmitters to be released into the synapse. The neurotransmitters carry the message to the next neuron, or "downstream" neuron, by physically docking at special sites called receptors. Like a car, the brain has both "accelerator" neurotransmitters, which prod a receiving neuron to fire, and "brake" neurotransmitters, which create the opposite effect. The brain needs both to run properly. Dozens of neurotransmitters have been identified, and each works in a different way from the others or on different parts of the brain. This turns out to be very helpful for scientists looking for ways to treat anxiety and depression — if only a few neurotransmitters existed and they worked on the entire brain, changing the activity of a particular neurotransmitter would have global — and probably undesirable — effects. But because so many neurotransmitters exist, and the receptors to which they attach themselves come in so many varieties, it's possible to develop drugs that target one certain receptor and thereby tweak the brain's machinery in relatively specific — and safe — ways.

Our ability to manipulate the brain has become more sophisticated in the past few decades, thanks to the explosion of new knowledge about how the brain works. For example, scientists in the 1960s were learning about the synapse and how neurotransmitter levels there affect disorders such as anxiety and depression. They learned that after a neurotransmitter molecule docks at a receptor on the "downstream" neuron, it is inactivated by enzymes or by special "reuptake" pumps that suck the neurotransmitter back into the sending axon. Drugs that block the enzymes or the reuptake pumps could alter neurotransmitter levels in the synapse, and that effect was found to alleviate anxiety or depression in some people.

In the 1970s and 1980s, attention shifted to the receptors themselves. It became clear that the different types of receptors made even more specific interventions possible, and some of the antidepressant drugs now on the market specifically target some receptors. In the past two decades scientific attention has shifted again to what happens *after* a receptor has been stimulated by a neurotransmitter. Receptors are like locks in the outside wall of a neuron. Neurotransmitter "keys" can cause the receptor "locks" to do a wide range of things, such as opening a brief hole in the cell membrane to allow chemicals to pass through or setting off cascades of further chemical reactions inside the receiving neuron. Sometimes these secondary signals reach all the way to the cell's genes, turning some on or off. The new field of research on so-called second messengers has opened up dozens of new potential targets for therapeutic drugs and promises both a better understanding of the mechanisms underlying disease and better drugs to alleviate symptoms.

But neurons, synapses, and neurotransmitters are just the fundamental working units of the brain — a little like transistors in a computer, only more elegantly complicated. Neurons, in turn, are linked together in vast circuits, and these circuits are assembled into discrete brain structures that specialize in different tasks, such as interpreting visual images, regulating heartbeat, or monitoring what all the other circuits are doing. The circuits that relate to anxiety and depression regulate the overall arousal level of the brain, generate emotions, and coordinate and monitor overall behavior. Use a sophisiticated scan to examine the brain of an anxious or depressed person, and you will see that parts of that brain are either underactive or overactive, compared with the brain of a person who is not anxious or depressed.[4] Those changes represent the collective quiescence or hyperactivity of vast webs of neurons, their synapses, and the neurotransmitters at work in those synapses. Both medications and psychotherapy can shift brain activity toward a healthier, more balanced configuration.

Underlying this phenomenon is the brain's plasticity, or malleability. Contrary to previous notions that the brain remains stable over the years and cannot grow new neurons, research now reveals that the brain is literally never the same from moment to moment. Not only are new neural connections constantly being formed, but entirely new neurons can grow — at least in certain regions such as the hippocampus, which is vital for memory formation. Memories and all other mental capacities work on a "use it or lose it" basis. When neurons fire together, they wire together, and the more they fire, the stronger the physical interrelationship grows. In a very real sense the brain is like a muscle, and that means we have the power to sculpt the brain over time in positive ways that leave us less vulnerable to anxiety and depression.

Progress in understanding the brain and the specific neural dysfunctions that can attend anxiety disorders or depression may lead to changes in the labels we use. The "bible" of psychiatric diagnosis is the *Diagnostic and Statistical Manual,* which is periodically revised by the American Psychiatric Association in light of new research, theories, and ideas. The current version is the *DSM-IV-TR* (the *TR* stands for "Text Revision"), but work is under way on the *DSM-V,* and a new set of labels may accompany its publication (not expected for several years as we write this book). The basic categories of anxiety disorders and depressive disorders are unlikely to change, but a new group of mixed-symptom disorders may be included. In addition, a more refined diagnostic framework may be introduced, to include information about a patient's genes, neurobiology, behavior, life situation and history, and response to treatments.[5] The inclusion of genetics and detailed neurobiology may produce a finer division of psychiatric disorders, allowing doctors to better predict which therapies, medications, or lifestyle changes would most likely work for a given patient — welcome progress indeed.

2

BUILDING EMOTIONAL
RESILIENCE

I bend and I break not.
— JEAN DE LA FONTAINE, *Fables*

FOR A LONG TIME, people have thought that the goals of treating anxiety or depression consist of eliminating unwanted or dysfunctional symptoms and restoring "normal" functioning. But progress in both psychology and neuroscience makes a more ambitious goal possible: the development of psychological resilience and emotional fitness.

This may sound overly optimistic. Shouldn't we be content to help a morose, physically weakened, and possibly suicidal person regain his or her health, equilibrium, and former outlook? Shouldn't we be satisfied to regain our old selves after suffering from anxiety or depression?

Good treatment can lead to far more than that. We must treat these disorders, of course, but we should also help people, whenever possible, to move beyond "recovery" to levels of functioning that are higher and more positive than those that existed before the disorder set in.

A key concept in this new perspective on human development is resilience: the capacity to maintain, recover, and improve mental and physical health in the face of challenge. The inclusion of both mental and physical health in the concept of resilience reflects the inseparability of mind and body. Physical health and mental health support each other and must be jointly considered during and after formal treatment for anxiety or depression.

Recent studies have shown that resilience can be improved with intentional effort. People can learn to build their psychological reserves, toughen their physical responses to stress, and become less vulnerable to anxiety or depression. And the lessons of resilience are as pertinent for "normal" people as for those struggling with anxiety or depression. Almost everyone can increase his resilience in some aspect of his physical or mental life.

Of course, being resilient doesn't mean never feeling bad nor having an invulnerable personality — far from it. The central metaphor of resilience is flexibility, not rigidity. Resilience implies a capacity to absorb blows, not repel them with armor. Resilience means having the full spectrum of human emotion, from positive to negative, as appropriate for a given situation, so that one does not become stuck in an emotion or fixated on a problem or event. This idea is hardly new, of course. Lao Tzu, the great Chinese philosopher, wrote something similar some twenty-six hundred years ago:

> Green plants are tender and filled with sap
> At their death they are withered and dry
> Therefore the stiff and unbending is the disciple of death
> The gentle and yielding is the disciple of life

A STORY OF RESILIENCE

Tho-van Tran seems to live a normal life. She's almost forty and has two school-age children, a husband, and a steady job in Bethesda, Maryland. But the path to her current life was anything but typical, and the laughter that punctuates her retelling of the journey suggests an unusual resilience of character.

Tho-van was born and raised in Saigon (now Ho Chi Minh City), in Vietnam. Her father, educated in France, ran a large bank. French was her first language, she went to a private school, and she led a relatively sheltered, upper-class life despite the war that raged during most of her childhood.

Then, on April 30, 1975, the South Vietnamese government surrendered to the North, and everything changed. Tho-van was twelve, and suddenly she had to adapt to a government that scorned her class.

"For us it was a change of life overnight," Tho-van says. "French school stopped. Our cars were taken. One of my uncles was put in jail. My brother was sent to the countryside to dig canals and irrigation ditches. The girls had to go out and collect cans and plastic bags, clean up trash."

For three years the family remained in Vietnam. But then her older brother was nearing the end of high school, and he was told he would be forcibly enrolled in the army and sent to Cambodia to be, in Tho-van's words, a "human shield."

The only way out of Vietnam at that time was by boat — a desperately risky undertaking. Pirates regularly seized boats of refugees, robbing, raping, and killing them. Storms sent hundreds to their deaths. The available boats were typically decaying and skippered by inexperienced men. But this was the only option for Tho-van's father and his family. For each of the sixteen family members who wanted to leave, he paid the government fifteen ounces of gold, a small fortune. The family was left with little money and almost no possessions.

"When we left, we wore two pairs of pants and two shirts," Tho-van says. "We had only one small bag each, and most of that was filled with powdered milk for the children, because we had no food, only water."

Tho-van's family was stuffed onto a small fishing boat with 242 other people, and they set off. They thought they were going to Thailand, but the "organizer" decided to go to Australia, which was absurdly far away.

On their first night on the open ocean, a storm churned the seas. One person was swept overboard; the rest were drenched and cold. The engine failed but was restored by a mechanic who happened to be among the boat people. The navigation system failed. The second-in-command took charge and made for Malaysia, the closest safe harbor.

After a week of crossing the South China Sea, with no food for any passengers, the boat was finally allowed to dock at the coastal Malaysian town of Kota Bharu — after everyone paid the local authority for the privilege. Eventually the International Red Cross was notified, and everyone was herded onto a bus and taken by boat to the island of Pula Tanga. When they got there, they had to build their own shelter.

"Nobody knew how to build a house," Tho-van says. "We would find a tree, cut it down, roll it down the hill, dig the sand up, stick the tree in, and tie the trees together. At one point two of my cousins and my brother climbed up on top while they were trying to put the roof up, and one cousin couldn't get down. It was funny. Here we were — we had lost everything, we were homeless, we were on an island, but instead of being sad, we're laughing."

After three months, a representative from France came to the island, and because Tho-van's family had relatives there, arrangements were made for them to emigrate to France. What followed were years of odd jobs for her father, schooling for Tho-van, moving from place to place, and eventually emigration to the United States, where one of her uncles owned a Vietnamese grocery store in Silver Spring, Maryland.

The driving force behind all the moves was family reunification. "We wanted to stay together and regroup with our grandmother in the United States," Tho-van says. "That's why I made the decision to come here from France. And my grandmother sponsored me. I was the first one of the family to come here. When my grandmother was getting older and sick, my parents came, and my brother came last."

At first Tho-van worked in the grocery store, despite her degree in accounting. Once the store began to succeed, she took a bank job and quickly rose to the position of assistant treasurer. By then she had married and had two young children. Again, family came first. "I had made a career in that small savings and loan," she says, "but after a while I didn't see my children anymore, so I resigned the position."

Later, her husband, a computer specialist at the National Institute of Mental Health, saw a job posting for a secretarial position there. It offered less pay and status than Tho-van had at the bank, but she took it because her supervisor gave her the flexibility she needed to care for her children.

Tho-van remembers her past clearly and unflinchingly. "Somehow, I was blessed to be able to adapt to different situations," she says. "You know, a lot of people would be depressed with losing everything, but somehow we managed. It was like, 'Okay, that's what it is.' We understood that we were lucky not to be in prison. I guess I inherited that ability to smile — most likely from my mother . . . she always laughs. She was always upbeat; somehow even in the hardest times I never saw her cry. Never. I think we learned the facts of life and the value of life quicker than a lot of younger kids. I guess I look on the good side. Thank God. If I looked on the other side, I'd probably cry."

Ordinary Magic

Child psychologist Ann Masten, of the University of Minnesota, calls resilience "ordinary magic." She says, "Resilience does not come from rare and special qualities, but from the everyday magic of ordinary human resources in the minds, brains, and bodies of children, in their families and relationships, and in their communities."[1]

We can see that in Tho-van's story. Her resilient spirit undoubtedly has genetic roots, but it also certainly relates to her upbringing by caring parents, physical health, belief in the value of traditions and family, and extremely strong family and community bonds.

The message, as true for children as for adults, is that resilience has many roots — it emerges from strength at four primary levels: biological, psychological, social, and external. When these pillars are strong, a distinctive cluster of personality traits appears: good intellectual functioning, effective self-regulation of emotions, positive self-concept, optimism, altruism, an active style of coping with stressful situations, and an ability to bond with a group for a common mission.

Resilience is not an all-or-nothing proposition, however. People are complicated, and so is their resilience. Some people have extraordinary resilience in one type of situation (such as being in physical danger) but not in another (such as dealing with emotional abuse). But the four pillars of resilience can be harnessed to maintain emotional fitness in the face of different types of challenges.

Physical health is the first pillar of resilience. One can seldom cope optimally with adversity, loss, or trauma if one is sick or incapacitated with an injury or chronic illness. Of course, as we just noted, no single factor is all-powerful, and this concept applies here. Some people who are very sick or battling a chronic illness such as cancer can be nonetheless impressively resilient in other ways, and this capacity supports them despite physical weakness.

Researchers have begun to link specific biological factors, such as levels of the stress hormone cortisol and the sex hormone testosterone, to resilience.[2] No single factor alone will greatly change one's resilience, but different factors combine to powerfully influence how sensitive one is to stress or threats, how quickly one's body calms down when a threat has passed, and how much stress and strain one's body and mind can bear.

Researchers are finding ways to accurately measure the biological dimension of resilience in order to develop a single "physical resilience number." For example, Teresa Seeman and her colleagues at UCLA developed a method of summing ten physiological markers of stress to arrive at a single measure that predicted resistance to stress-related diseases in a group of older adults.[3] Such attempts provide models to measure resilience; in the future, people may receive a resilience measure along with reports of blood pressure and cholesterol level during regular medical exams. Such an assessment could help clinicians identify those at risk for anxiety or depression following stress or trauma and would allow people to monitor their own physical resilience over time.

Genes certainly play a role in setting broad limits on one's biological resilience, but genes are not destiny. You may be stuck with your eye color, but you are not stuck with a given level of resilience. Regardless of age or physical condition, people can improve their resilience by taking simple steps such as eating well, exercising, getting enough sleep, and avoiding excessive use of alcohol and other recreational drugs. Aerobic exercise, for instance, reduces cortisol, raises testosterone, improves insulin function, and alters a variety of brain chemicals in ways that improve mood.[4]

The second pillar is psychological resilience, which arises from the quality of one's upbringing, one's capacity to balance emotion and reason, and the depth of meaning one finds in life. Psychological resilience is closely tied to biological resilience, a relationship that researchers are now actively exploring in the new field of social cognition — the intersection of neuroscience and sociology.[5] But it also is powerfully related to external factors. For example, many studies have proved the vital importance of emotional closeness and attachment in the development of psychological health — particularly during the earliest years of life. The ideas of John Bowlby, a pioneering researcher into attachment, remain as valid today as they were in the 1950s, when he was working: "A central feature of my concept of parenting is the provision by both parents of a secure base from which a child or an adolescent can make sorties into the outside world and to which he can return knowing for sure that he will be welcomed when he gets there, nourished physically and emotionally, comforted if distressed, reassured if frightened."[6]

Having (or providing) ample opportunities for emotional bonding and attachment builds an important foundation for later resilience. Maintaining physical contact, developing trust, fostering self-confidence and self-esteem, providing stable surroundings, and establishing open and effective communication between parents and children all contribute to resilience.

Of course, psychological health and resilience can also be impaired during development by physical, emotional, or sexual abuse, neglect, inconsistent expectations, and a host of other traumas. Fortunately, such stressors are usually not crippling if the traumatizing events end and children come under competent care. In the 1990s, for instance, the British researcher Michael Rutter conducted extensive work with orphans in Romania who were neglected by state-run institutions. He found that the orphans showed some long-lasting and irreversible brain damage due to their neglect but that they were also remarkably able to recover if adopted and raised by healthy parents.[7]

A feature of psychological resilience is the capacity to view events in ways that promote effective coping. In psychological terms, this is called appraisal. Different people may view, or appraise, a given event quite differently, which can have far-reaching implications. Generally speaking, adverse events can be viewed as either threats or challenges.

If a situation is appraised as a threat, the body reacts immediately. A cascade of hormones, including adrenaline and cortisol, surge through the body, preparing it for action. Meanwhile, on an emotional level, an appraisal of threat elicits fear, apprehension, anxiety, and defensiveness. Situations viewed as challenges, however, have quite different hormonal and emotional qualities. Challenge implies the possibility for growth or gain, and the emotions surrounding a challenge are often positive: eagerness, excitement, and determination, for example. The hormones released by an appraisal of challenge include growth factors, insulin, and other compounds that promote cell repair, trigger relaxation responses, and stimulate efficient energy use.[8]

Both types of appraisal can be valid, and both types of hormonal response can be helpful. After all, life sometimes presents threats, and our emotional and physical responses help us meet them. But people who habitually or unconsciously assess situations as threats will erode their resilience by constantly engaging defensive bodily responses, which are biologically taxing.

Of course, sometimes a situation involves both threatening and challenging aspects. A new job opportunity may offer potential for gains in status and money but also the threat of failure and loss. This blended outlook is embodied in the Chinese word for crisis: *wei ji*, which translates as "dangerous opportunity."

As long as a balance exists between these opposing hormonal responses, and as long as the threat or stressor is not constant or chronic, exposure to threats can actually toughen the hormonal response system and confer greater resilience. The trouble comes when a nonthreatening event, such as constructive criticism, is appraised as a threat rather than a challenge, or when an actual threat is unrelenting, as in the case of long-term child abuse by a parent or sibling.

Psychological resilience is also related to the sturdiness of one's worldview and the quality of one's fundamental assumptions. Sometimes situations arise that shake the foundations of what we assumed was true about our lives, our world, and our place in the cosmos. We discover an affair. A parent dies unexpectedly. A friend commits suicide. Terrorism strikes with a magnitude and proximity we never imagined. The shattering of basic assumptions leaves one vulnerable to depression, anxiety, or both.

Psychologists such as Ronnie Janoff-Bulman at the University of Massachusetts–Amherst have found that people construct worldviews by making generalizations based on usually positive early experiences. They resist changing these ideas even in the face of contradictory evidence.[9] Such stubbornness concerning fundamental beliefs can be good in moderation, but clinging to a core worldview based on childhood generalizations can, in the context of a traumatic event, leave one vulnerable to disorientation, confusion, or more serious psychological problems. On the other hand, basic assumptions that have evolved to accommodate the sometimes harsh realities of life improve resilience. The unexpected death of a loved one, for example, may still be shocking and produce gut-wrenching sadness, but the experience will not feel as dire or fundamentally threatening as it would for someone who never truly considered an unexpected death to be really possible.

The last component of psychological resilience arises from having a sense of meaning in life. As Sigmund Freud noted, "Men are strong as long as they stand for an idea." Viktor Frankl, a renowned psychiatrist and Holocaust survivor, wrote that "meaning is found in serving a cause or pursuing a vocation or mission in life — endeavors that have an inspiring or uplifting effect on us."[10]

Whether one finds personal meaning in spiritual or secular beliefs is irrelevant. What matters is having a useful and meaningful role in life, particularly one that involves helping others. Having a mission or goal larger than oneself can provide a long-term view that helps keep daily frustrations, losses, or problems in perspective. Helping others appears to bolster one's own capacity to withstand stress or trauma, a phenomenon noted in World War II among citizens caring for others after air raids in London. Another example comes from researchers who find that when people who suffer from specific fears are asked to help others with similar concerns, their own level of fear decreases.[11]

Psychological resilience relates to the third pillar of resilience: one's social world. All primates are intensely social creatures, and humans are the most socially complex of all. We have a deep instinct to form groups, create social hierarchies, bond emotionally, and simply hang out together. Having a network of friends and family is a powerful safety net in times of trouble and a key factor in resilience.[12] Particularly important are confiding relationships — connections secure enough to sustain disclosure of a person's deepest feelings, most embarrassing traits, or worst problems. Talking to somebody (or writing about it to yourself) can allow you to step back and take a wider perspective — and, of course, a confidant may provide some helpful ideas or emotional support as well.

Of course, talking about sensitive or traumatic issues should always be voluntary. Forcing another person to talk about something in the belief that the catharsis will be good for him or her is always a mistake and can be quite harmful. But at the right time and place, sharing difficult or painful truths about one's life can be tremendously helpful or healing.

The last pillar of resilience is one's set of external supports, such as money, education, food, clothing, and shelter. In general, having such supports contributes only modestly to resilience, but lacking them significantly erodes it. For example, many studies show that wealth beyond that needed for adequate shelter, food, and opportunity does little to increase happiness.[13] But having money can help in times of crisis by allowing one freedom, for example, to hire others to do household work or take a trip to visit family members who can provide comfort and support. Similarly, having a college education by itself doesn't guarantee resilience, but it does confer some protection, perhaps because education develops "cognitive complexity," a variety of intellectual abilities and the capacity to view matters from multiple perspectives. Still, in many ways, the external components of resilience are the least important of the factors we've just discussed.

The four pillars of resilience combine and change to create one's overall level of resilience at any given time. Investigators in this field refer to the sum of physical, emotional, and mental stressors in life as one's "allostatic load." This load is always in flux — sometimes high, sometimes low. The related term *allostasis* means "maintaining mental and physical stability by changing in response to circumstances." Allostasis requires continual adjustments and alterations in one's internal and external world in response to constantly changing conditions. A simple example is the way heart rate varies during exercise. But the same type of dynamic works at a psychological level as well — one can adjust beliefs, priorities, goals, and strategies in response to a changing allostatic load. This is the hallmark of resilience: the ability to smoothly adjust to the demands of the outside world to maintain an optimal allostasis.

BECOMING MORE RESILIENT

Friedrich Nietzsche's famous quote, "What does not destroy me makes me strong," contains an important element of truth verified by researchers studying resilience. Many people emerge from a challenge, such as the loss of a loved one, sexual abuse, or combat, saying they have gained from their experience. Those who have struggled with anxiety or depression often report the same thing. When they are effectively treated, anxiety and depression can be transformative experiences. This is not to say that anybody would intentionally choose to experience a mood disorder as a pathway to personal growth; it is simply an acknowledgment that growth is a possible — indeed desirable — outcome of a struggle with a mood disorder.

Evidence for the potential positive value of adversity comes primarily from research not specifically focused on mood disorders, but the results are transferable and relevant. Examples reviewed in the book *Posttraumatic Growth* include the following:

- Rape victims who had experienced the loss of a significant person prior to their assault had fewer difficulties adjusting.
- Older adults are less subject to psychological impairment after natural disasters due to their greater recognition of personal vulnerability.
- Vietnam veterans who had a stressful childhood were less likely to develop posttraumatic stress disorder.[14]

Such research — and stories such as Tho-van's — suggests that adversity or trauma can sometimes produce greater resilience. For instance, in *Posttraumatic Growth* a woman with a painful chronic illness says: "Living with this disease has taught me so many precious things that I wouldn't have learned if I were healthy. I guess the most important things it has taught me are to appreciate what life can hold for you every day and to be grateful for the loving relationships in your life."[15]

Another positive effect of adversity is a purely physical toughening, which involves the body systems that release and regulate cortisol and other hormones during stressful or threatening situations — the so-called fight-or-flight system. Some military training techniques that prepare soldiers for hazardous or unexpected conditions are based on this principle. The goal is to train both the mind and the fight-or-flight system to respond appropriately to acute danger and then to quickly dampen the response once danger has passed. The general principle is widely applicable, however. On first exposure to a stressor, a person experiences a large stress-hormone response, which triggers a host of bodily changes, ranging from a racing heart and sweaty palms to nausea and pallor. If, after a period of rest, the stressor is repeated, the hormonal spike is lower — the system has adapted to the stress and become less sensitive. It has grown tougher. This adaptation has also been called "stress inoculation" because the exposure to intermittent stress "inoculates" a person against further stress.

Recent research suggests that aerobic exercise can produce toughening effects that mirror those induced by moderate, intermittent stress. For example, physical training programs have been linked to lower baseline physiological arousal rates, quicker return to baseline after stress, improved use of blood sugar, reduction in muscle tension, and a reduction in various compounds associated with the fight-or-flight arousal of the nervous system.[16]

The bottom line is that practically everyone can become tougher, more resilient, and less vulnerable to mood disorders or anxiety. The following suggestions for doing so are organized according to the hierarchy of human needs pointed out decades ago by the psychologist Abraham Maslow. He noted that fundamental needs, such as food and shelter, must be addressed before dealing with higher-level needs such as security, love, or creativity. In the same way, the first suggestions on the following list should be tackled before moving on to higher-level factors for increasing resilience, such as creating or maintaining confiding relationships. This isn't a hard-and-fast rule — you can improve your physical health at the same time you work on finding meaning in your life, for instance — it's just a general theme to keep in mind as you work to raise your resilience.

- **TREAT ANY EXISTING PHYSICAL OR MENTAL ILLNESS.** A serious physical or mental condition such as poorly managed diabetes or untreated depression makes it harder to improve resilience. Even a minor illness is disruptive and energy-draining, and it steals pleasure and satisfaction from life. Physical health promotes resilience — and improving resilience promotes physical health.

- TREAT EXISTING SUBSTANCE ABUSE OR ADDICTION PROBLEMS. Habitual or addictive use of alcohol and other drugs can directly destabilize the biological factors, mentioned earlier, that regulate physical resilience. Substance abuse and addiction can also, of course, wreak havoc on relationships, careers, and other important building blocks of resilience.

- EXERCISE AND EAT RIGHT. Most people know they should exercise at least thirty minutes a day and eat a diet high in fruits and vegetables and low in refined sugar and saturated fat, so we won't belabor this point. Just remember that resilience resides in your cells, organs, and immune system as much as in your psychology, family, and life circumstances.

- TAKE TIME OFF. As mentioned previously, mild to moderate stress can actually strengthen physical resilience as long as you give your body time to recover. Unremitting stress, however, weakens the body, reduces resilience, and may make you more vulnerable to future stressors.

- ESTABLISH OR PRESERVE AT LEAST ONE CONFIDING RELATIONSHIP. Establishing a relationship in which painful or embarrassing situations can be shared takes time, energy, and a willingness to listen as well as talk. Of course, in order to confide something to somebody else, you first have to confide it to yourself. Admitting to our own foibles, failures, losses, and pain is never easy, but it's the first step to an honest and satisfying relationship with someone else.

- CHALLENGE YOURSELF. Resilience is fostered by setting goals and working hard to achieve them. By leaving your "comfort zone" in any endeavor and risking short-term failure for long-term success, you can gain confidence, mastery, and added strength.

- LOOK FOR MEANING. People discover meaning in their lives in many ways, but a common outcome is becoming involved in a cause, idea, or activity larger than themselves. It doesn't matter if one's motivation is secular or spiritual — what counts is engaging with others in something you care about deeply. Those connections and the shared sense of mission involved are important elements of resilience.

Becoming a more resilient person is rarely a smooth, uninterrupted process. Life events will happen that sometimes support and occasionally erode resilience. You may get promoted, find a loving partner, or have a meaningful spiritual experience. You may also lose a loved one, become ill, or come under unusual stress from your job or family situation. The key is to maintain as much progress as possible, understanding that resilience doesn't mean freedom from pain but rather that life's inevitable pain will not so overwhelm you that you slip into disorders such as anxiety and depression.

3

MOOD AND
PHYSICAL HEALTH

When the mind is upset by some overwhelming fear, we see all the
spirit in every limb upset in sympathy.

— LUCRETIUS, 55 B.C.E.

IT WAS SOMETIME AFTER LUNCH on a Friday in the autumn of 2000
that Carter (a pseudonym), a thirty-six-year-old graphic designer, first noticed an odd tingling pain in his chin.

"I just thought, okay, something's going on . . . Maybe what I ate had
gone bad," he says. "I took some aspirin and lay down, thinking it would go
away. But I couldn't sleep, and lying down made the pain more intense."

Carter had moved to Massachusetts from Pasadena only three weeks
previously to live with his fiancée. He hadn't yet begun to look for work
and was home alone.

After about three hours the tingling pain began to spread from his
chin to his jaw, and he began to worry. He searched the Internet for information, but the only physical problem that seemed to fit his symptoms was
a heart attack, which he thought was impossible. As he kept reading, he
broke out in a cold sweat. Then he read that another common heart-attack
symptom is an unexplainable sense of doom. Yes, he thought to himself . . .
that's it. A sense of doom. He got up and drove to the nearest hospital.
Waves of nausea forced him to stop along the way to vomit.

Initially, the attending doctors did not think Carter had heart disease.
He was young, didn't smoke, didn't drink, and wasn't overweight. All their
tests were inconclusive; but the chin and jaw pain were just as intense, even
after placing a nitroglycerin pill under his tongue. Finally, a blood test for
a specific compound released by damaged heart muscle confirmed that
Carter was experiencing a heart attack.

"It was devastating, unbelievable," he recalls. "I thought this shouldn't
be happening to me. Maybe at sixty-six, but not thirty-six."

Carter's blocked coronary artery was widened with balloon angio-plasty, and a tiny wire-mesh tube called a stent was implanted to prop open the artery. Soon he was back home, where he received supportive cards, calls, letters, and emails.

Later Carter celebrated Thanksgiving with his fiancée's family, yet the holiday poignantly reminded him of his isolation from friends, the delay in his career ambitions, and the changes wrought by the heart attack, such as his doctor's order not to drive for six weeks.

"I felt as though I was never going to be the same person again," he says. "I felt emasculated, robbed of a sense of security that I'd taken for granted. And I knew I'd forever be looking over my shoulder, wondering not if but when it would happen again."

Carter was sinking into depression. "I began to doubt my own self-worth or whether I could even work again because of the stress involved," he says. "I retreated by sleeping a lot. And worst of all, I started fighting with my fiancée. She's such a wonderful person. She's got the biggest heart in the world and wanted desperately to help me, and she couldn't. I didn't want her help."

Around the turn of the year Carter had given up on himself, and his thoughts turned to suicide — specifically, while driving. Whether prompted by those deadly thoughts, his fiancée's pressure on him to get help, or just his own realization that he was in serious trouble, he finally went to see a therapist. He was prescribed an antidepressant and began intensive twice-weekly therapy sessions.

"I'd say the psychotherapy was more important than the medication," he says. "The medication helped me with my therapeutic work — I would have been unresponsive, a lump on a log without it — but the medication couldn't complete the work. That was my job."

In April he began to look for work, and a month later he was doing freelance design for a nearby college. Soon they hired him full-time. He and his fiancée began planning a fall wedding. Feeling good, he stopped taking his medication and ended therapy, thinking he had accomplished the work he wanted.

Three weeks before the wedding, Carter felt the same tingling sensation in his chin. Another artery had become almost totally blocked. He and his fiancée acted fast, and they made it to the hospital before serious damage was done. Still, they postponed the wedding, and a new round of rehab and recovery ensued. Once again, Carter became depressed, but this time he didn't wait to begin the medication and therapy, and he never hit bottom.

A year and a half later, Carter is sitting outside his office, talking about it all. He and his fiancée got married the following spring. He hasn't had another heart attack. He enjoys his work but doesn't keep his former work-aholic pace. He feels healthy. But he doesn't take much for granted any-more.

"I don't shy away from the shadows," he says. "They're there. But I'm aware of them, aware of depression, of its effects and of its treatment. That awareness is so key. I realized that I don't have to be depressed the rest of my life. Sure, I have 'normal' depressed times, but that's okay. I accept that. Mostly I'm just happy to be here."

The Mind-Body Connection

In recent years research findings have steadily piled up confirming the age-old idea that the connection between mind and body is a two-way street. Like Carter, you may certainly get depressed, for instance, from the experi-ence of a serious illness such as a heart attack.

But we also now know that the reverse is also true: being depressed raises the risk for a host of illnesses. The exact biological mechanisms behind such links are the subject of intense scrutiny right now, and the full answers are not yet in. But we already know enough to add urgency to the goal of treating anxiety and depression as quickly and effectively as possible.

It's easy to say that the mind and the body are connected — it's even a commonplace notion in some circles, such as the holistic health commu-nity. But it is not immediately obvious *how*, in fact, the two are connected. The mind, after all, is nonmaterial — an almost ghostlike entity somehow produced by our brains. How can something as seemingly evanescent as a mood possibly affect something physical like a blood vessel?

First of all, just because the mind is nonphysical doesn't mean it's not real. Such things as beauty, truth, and noon are all perfectly real, though immaterial. More important, the immaterial mind completely depends on the material brain for its existence and various properties. When you make a decision with your mind, vast networks of connected brain cells fire in a particular sequence. When you smell a rose, a constellation of brain cells lights up, and that constellation is connected to other physical networks that create and recall memory. When you see a snake, a part of the brain charged with detecting potentially dangerous images explodes with activity and produces the feelings that another part of the brain interprets as fear. Immaterial moods arise from material brain changes, and scientists are now linking those changes to physical health.

The brain is directly connected to the body via the nervous system, which radiates from the spinal cord to practically every cell. In addition, the brain indirectly influences the body by telling various organs to either increase or decrease hormone levels. Adrenaline, cortisol, estrogen, testosterone, insulin, and dozens of other hormones powerfully affect the cardiovascular and immune systems as well as metabolism, alertness, and a host of other functions.

The neurotransmitters (described in Chapter 1) are also used by nerve cells throughout the body and can directly affect physiology. Serotonin, for example, which is the neurotransmitter manipulated by Prozac (fluoxetine) and related antidepressants, not only regulates mood but also helps maintain the elasticity of blood vessels and thus affects blood pressure. That's where it gets its name: *sero* (Greek for "blood") and *tonin* (Greek for "tone" or "tension"). Serotonin also plays a critical role in blood platelets, which govern how quickly blood clots. Changing the level of any of the dozens of neurotransmitters, in other words, can affect both brain and body.

The connections between brain and body explain why a bodily illness, such as a cold, affects mood, thinking, and memory, and conversely, why treating a psychological condition can improve physical health. Mind and body are linked in many ways, but one of the best-studied is a stress-sensitive system called the hypothalamic-pituitary-adrenal axis (HPA axis for short). The hypothalamus is a brain region that controls a number of body systems such as temperature, appetite, and blood pressure. Stress or a perceived threat generates signals that stimulate the hypothalamus to release a chemical signal to the nearby pituitary gland. The pituitary, in turn, releases a powerful hormone that travels through the bloodstream to the adrenal glands on top of the kidneys. The hormones released by the adrenal glands can affect kidney function, blood-sugar level, the inflammatory response, immune function, heart rate, metabolism, and blood pressure.

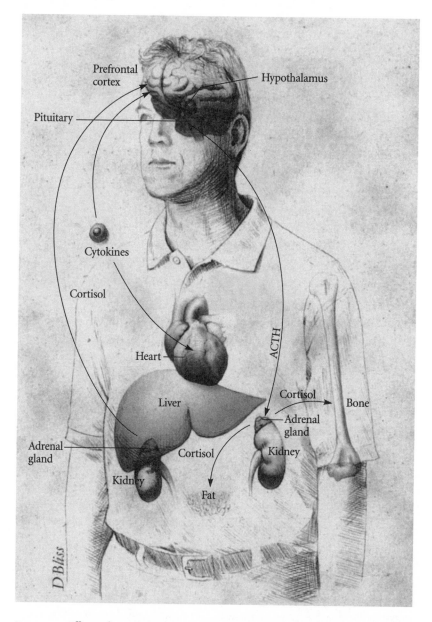

FIGURE 3. *Effects of mood changes on the body.* Moods or emotions can affect the body and vice versa. For example, stress or depression can stimulate the brain's hypothalamus to send a signal to the pituitary, the body's "master gland." The pituitary releases the hormone ACTH, which leads to the release of hormones such as cortisol from the adrenal glands, on top of the kidneys. Cortisol exerts many effects, such as increasing fat, reducing bone mass, and altering the function of brain areas such as the prefrontal cortex, which is critical to mood regulation, among other things. Depression can also increase levels of chemicals called cytokines, which can in turn raise the risk of clogging in the small arteries of the heart and brain. *American Journal of Psychiatry* 159 (2002): 11. Copyright 2000, the American Psychiatric Association. Reprinted with modifications by permission.

The loop is closed when the hormones released by the adrenal glands act on the hypothalamus to turn off the original signal. Anxiety and depression can create stress that shifts the HPA axis into overdrive and interferes with its ability to switch itself off when not needed. This, in turn, can lead to a host of malfunctions in the cardiovascular, immune, and metabolic systems.

Immune system changes are particularly important. Chronic HPA-axis activation reduces the activity of certain cells in the immune system that help kill viruses, bacteria, and worn-out cells. Ever more research is linking major diseases with anxiety, depression, or both. In some cases, such as heart disease, research shows that a psychiatric disorder, depression, markedly increases the risk for disease. In other cases, such as cancer, the mental dysfunction is more often a result of the disease. In either case, spotting and quickly treating anxiety and depression help prevent further illness and speed healing.

HEART DISEASE AND STROKE

First, consider the connections between anxiety, depression, and heart disease, which is the leading cause of death in the United States, killing nearly a million people here each year.[1] Millions of survivors end up burdened by anxiety, depression, or both. For example, one study found that a third of heart-attack survivors become depressed within a year.[2]

Such depression takes a heavy toll. Compared with nondepressed patients, depressed patients with heart disease return to work more slowly, are more likely to be rehospitalized or die, and incur higher costs for their medical care.[3]

Exactly why heart disease increases the risk of depression (and perhaps anxiety) is not yet known. The stress, fear, and uncertainty surrounding a heart attack or other heart condition can certainly precipitate depressed mood and a range of anxiety symptoms.[4] And it could be that some problems that affect the heart also affect the brain. The fatty deposits that clog coronary arteries, for example, may also clog tiny arteries in the brain, leading to "micro-strokes" that impair mood without otherwise being noticed.

Depression, in turn, raises the risk of heart disease — as much as four times that of nondepressed people.[5] Also, anxiety and depression may promote unhealthful behaviors such as eating high-fat foods, smoking or drinking to excess, and not exercising. Depression, and possibly anxiety, has also been shown to increase the stickiness of the blood and the speed with which it clots, both of which raise the risk for a heart attack or stroke. Depression also seems to interfere with the heart's ability to respond quickly to changes in oxygen demand — so-called heart-rate variability. Finally, depression dampens the immune system, which makes it harder for the body to clear fat from coronary blood vessels.

Several studies have shown that depression can be safely and effectively treated in patients with heart disease.[6] That's good news because so many people have suffered without recognition or adequate treatment of their symptoms. Whether alleviating depression improves the survival and overall health of heart-disease patients is being actively investigated. The most recent study compared two groups of male and female heart-attack survivors: one group got regular cardiac care, and the other got psychotherapy and/or antidepressants.[7] After six months those getting the extra help were significantly less depressed than were the members of the control group. But after two years, no differences between the two groups were found in overall survival or rates of second heart attacks. This result should be interpreted cautiously, however, because, for ethical reasons, about 20 percent of those in the "untreated" group actually did get antidepressant therapy.

More studies are under way to explore this issue, but in the meantime it makes sense to watch closely for signs of emotional disorders in heart-disease patients and to see that these illnesses are treated quickly. Sadly, many such patients are not getting the help they need with mood disorders. In the most recent study to look into the matter, only one in four depressed cardiac patients received treatment.[8] What is clear is that treating depression in patients with heart disease with antidepressants is safe and effective.

Related to heart disease is stroke — brain damage caused by a blocked or ruptured cerebral artery. About one in every five people who suffer a stroke experience full-blown depression, which translates to 120,000 people each year.[9] Untreated, depression in stroke victims typically lasts a year. Among the factors that affect the likelihood and severity of depression following a stroke are the location of the brain injury, previous or family history of depression, and how the person functioned socially before the stroke.

Depression among stroke victims is underdiagnosed because so many of its symptoms resemble symptoms of stroke, such as lethargy, appetite changes, and sleep disruption. Caregivers must be alert to signs of anxiety and depression because effective treatment is likely to speed the recovery from the stroke itself. A 2003 study by Robert Robinson of the University of Iowa showed that treating depression in people who had a stroke improved their ability to perform tasks of daily living as well as enhancing their thinking and memory.[10]

CHRONIC DISEASES AND PAIN

Anxiety and depression are also associated with a number of chronic diseases such as diabetes, which afflicts at least 16 million people in the United States.[11] Although any chronic disease is associated with an increased prevalence of mood disorders, diabetes is unusually challenging because the burden of care falls primarily on the individual. The job can be tough, and difficulties with disease management can lead to depression. Several studies suggest that diabetes doubles the risk of depression compared to those without the disorder.[12] Conversely, depression can make diabetes worse by, for example, decreasing the body's sensitivity to insulin, which makes it harder to keep blood-sugar levels normal. Fortunately, this negative feedback loop can be interrupted. Good treatment of diabetes can directly help with the depression: keeping blood-sugar levels under control, eating a healthful diet, exercising regularly, and getting enough sleep can all improve a person's mood and reduce the symptoms of anxiety and depression.

Depression, and possibly anxiety, also raises one's risk for the bone-wasting disease osteoporosis.[13] Osteoporosis, in turn, contributes to thousands of deaths each year by making people vulnerable to hip fractures, which, in older adults, can result in long-term hospitalization and a rapid decline in health. The higher levels of cortisol and lower levels of growth hormone that can accompany depression probably play a role in this increased risk. It's also likely that the lack of energy and motivation typical of depression leads people to exercise less and eat a less healthful diet; both behaviors can speed osteoporosis.

The implications are particularly serious for women because they are diagnosed with depression twice as often as men and are five times more likely than men to have osteoporosis.[14] (Other risk factors for osteo-porosis include preexisting low bone density, a family history of osteoporosis, a previous fracture, thinness, low calcium intake, and smoking.) In one study, seriously depressed women were more likely to fall and had more fractures than nondepressed women.[15] Women at risk for osteoporosis should consult their physicians and take steps to minimize or reverse bone loss, such as taking calcium supplements, exercising regularly, and, perhaps, taking a medication that targets osteoporosis. Given the research to date, these habits become all the more imperative if a woman is also depressed.

Thanks to progress in creating drugs to fight the human immunodeficiency virus (HIV), more and more people today are living for many years with AIDS, the disease caused by the virus. But like people who cope with other chronic diseases, those with HIV or AIDS have a higher risk of suffering from anxiety and depression. Some studies have also found that high stress and depressive symptoms are associated with a more rapid progression to AIDS among those infected with HIV. For example, researchers at the University of North Carolina School of Medicine found that in two groups of men with HIV but no symptoms, the probability of getting AIDS after five years was about two to three times higher among those who experienced above-average stress or who had below-average levels of social support.[16]

Although as many as one in three persons with HIV may suffer from depression, warning signs of anxiety or depression such as fatigue, sadness, or appetite changes are often attributed to HIV rather than to a mood disorder. People with HIV, their families and friends, and even their physicians may assume that depression is an inevitable reaction to being diagnosed with HIV. But as we've noted, anxiety and depression are not the same as transient or mild anxious or depressive moods and should be treated as vigorously as any other illness.

Treating depression helps people better manage AIDS, thus enhancing survival and quality of life. Like other people with chronic diseases, these patients need carefully considered treatment plans, including close attention to possible adverse reactions between medications.

Chronic pain, such as that from migraines or low-back injury, greatly raises the risk for depression and, probably, anxiety. A recent study of almost 19,000 people, published in 2003, found that almost half of those with major depression suffered from chronic pain.[17] Those with major depression were four times more likely than the nondepressed to suffer from joint, limb, or back pain; headaches; or gastrointestinal pain. Such findings are important because the presence of chronic pain is not on the standard checklist of symptoms for depression. Caregivers and patients themselves should be more alert to signs of depression so that proper treatment can be given. As mentioned earlier, pain and depression can form a feedback loop: the pain makes the depression worse, which makes the pain worse, and so on.

Treating the depression will certainly improve a patient's overall quality of life and is likely to reduce pain too. In fact, an older class of antidepressants called the tricyclics has been known to directly dampen pain. New clinical trials are testing a variety of depression treatments to see if they also reduce chronic pain. Meanwhile, we still recommend aggressive treatment of anxiety and depression for those with chronic pain because the disorders themselves are psychically painful and debilitating.

CANCER

Cancer can cause anxiety, depression, or both. Simply put, being diagnosed with cancer is upsetting and depressing. In addition, some of the drugs used to treat cancer make depression more likely — a situation that can sometimes be avoided with simultaneous use of an antidepressant.[18] (For details, see Appendix III.) Studies show that anywhere from one of every four to one of every five cancer patients reports mild or moderate depression. People who have the most serious pain and other symptoms are at highest risk.[19] In turn, anxiety and depression make it harder to perform basic life functions, increase pain intensity, and erode quality of life over the course of the illness. It is also frustratingly clear that these conditions are underdetected and undertreated, in part because both physicians and the family and friends of a cancer patient often view anxiety and depression as "normal" and in part because some symptoms of cancer (for instance, weight loss, lack of energy, and sleep disturbance) mimic signs of depression.[20] But spotting and treating anxiety and depression in cancer patients are critical because the mood disturbances and the disease symptoms can feed upon each other harmfully.

Although the link showing that cancer can precipitate anxiety and depression is clear, the reverse relationship is still the subject of debate. Some studies suggest that being anxious or depressed does not raise one's risk for cancer. For instance, one study found that the rate of depression among newly diagnosed cancer patients was similar to the rates among patients with other serious medical diagnoses.[21] This implies that depression was not a factor in whether or not the people in this study were diagnosed with cancer. On the other hand, other studies suggest that depression *does* increase the risk of cancer. Two recent studies found a modest, but significant, rise in the number of deaths from breast cancer among women who were seriously depressed.[22] One of the studies, a nationwide survey of women in Denmark, found that women with early-stage breast cancer have a slightly higher risk of dying from cancer if they suffer from depression after their diagnosis. Women with more serious late-stage cancer have a higher risk of dying if they suffered from depression *before* their diagnosis. Such findings are preliminary and suggest a connection between depression and the onset of cancer, but much work remains to determine precisely what those links might be. Given the immune system changes discussed earlier, anxiety and depression could plausibly alter one's vulnerability to cancer in complicated and subtle ways.[23]

OTHER CONDITIONS

Because we believe in making statements and claims only when they can be backed up by well-conducted studies, we have limited our discussion thus far to the conditions that have been most thoroughly studied. But we want to make clear that these are undoubtedly not the only physical conditions related to anxiety and depression. Preliminary evidence exists for a connection between anxiety and depression and the following conditions: ulcers, arthritis, high blood pressure, Parkinson disease, Alzheimer disease, asthma, and certain chronic stomach conditions.[24]

Of course, recognizing a potential connection between anxiety and depression and physical illness doesn't mean a mental dysfunction is *always* involved with a disease — and it certainly doesn't imply that patients should feel they are to blame, somehow, for an illness. Far from it! We simply want to reduce the levels of undetected anxiety and depression among the ill so they can recover faster and raise awareness about the role of anxiety and depression in illness to motivate people to seek help as quickly as possible.

PART II

Diagnosing and Finding Optimal Treatment for Anxiety and Depression

4

THE WORLD OF
ANXIETY DISORDERS

Worry gives a small thing a big shadow.

— Swedish proverb

IT WAS 1975, and Isaac (a pseudonym) was in eleventh grade, sitting in class as the teacher droned on. Suddenly his heart began to pound in his chest; he felt dizzy and short of breath.

"I had no idea what was happening," he says. "I got out of my chair and told the teacher I felt sick. I went into the hallway and sat down."

After about thirty minutes Isaac's pulse slowed and he could breathe easily again. Shaken and bewildered, he returned to class. A month later it happened again, out of the blue. Thinking he might have a heart problem, he went to his family doctor. After ruling out a heart condition, the doctor suggested Xanax (alprazolam), a fast-acting sedative often used to calm anxiety.

"It helped for a little while," he recalls. But as the years passed, the Xanax became progressively less effective. His doctor repeatedly raised the dose, but the attacks became more debilitating.

"I still had no idea what was going on," he said. "I actually thought I was going crazy. I'd go to the hospital and they'd do all these scans and say nothing was wrong. But I was still having the vertigo and the attacks. It got so that any situation in which I felt trapped would trigger an attack. I'd always drive with the windows open. Even being stuck at a red light would set me off, and I'd try to run the light so I didn't have to stop."

By this time Isaac was married with two young children and had a career as a portrait photographer. He struggled on in what became a daily battle to cope with the attacks.

By 1997 he was desperate.

"I was totally depressed," he says. "I felt terrible from all the anxiety and the panic attacks and all the stuff I couldn't do. I didn't want to go out of the house because I was afraid of what might happen. And the worrying . . . the constant worrying."

The anxiety frustrated his wife.

"It was confusing for her," Isaac says. "People can't understand what you're talking about. A person who hasn't gone through this can't comprehend the pain that anxiety can cause. I'd rather have physical pain than that kind of pain. I mean, if you break your arm or something, you know you broke your arm and it'll get better. With this . . . you don't know what's happening and you don't know if it'll be worse or better the next day."

Having read about an anxiety program at a university hospital two hours away from his home in South Carolina, Isaac ended up seeing a psychiatrist experienced with anxiety disorders. The psychiatrist put a definitive name on Isaac's condition — panic disorder — and explained the biological roots of the illness. Isaac recalled that his grandmother was anxious and always took what she called "nerve pills."

"Just knowing what was going on for the first time was a help," Isaac says. "Trying to figure it out on my own and not knowing were really hard. And you don't tell people about it because they look at you like you're really a crazy person."

But Isaac's path to wellness was no picnic. Because his brain and body had become used to the high doses of Xanax, his psychiatrist started to wean him off that drug while beginning treatment with an antidepressant known to reduce panic symptoms.

"At first I felt worse," Isaac says. "I called him back and said, 'You've got to be kidding. I can't take this.' But he told me to hang in there, that it was going to work, that it takes time."

For a month Isaac waited, feeling, he says, "like a zombie" and still having panic attacks. "And then, one morning I woke up and it was almost like a miracle. Out of the blue, I felt totally different. It's hard to explain, really."

Seven years have passed now since that transformative morning, and Isaac's life is more normal than it's been since his first panic attack in eleventh grade. He still does not like to drive over bridges — one of the things that used to trigger an attack — and he prefers not to fly if he can help it. He also, from time to time, has an attack, such as when he was at an amusement park and took a ride that confined him in a small, dark capsule. But now he knows what's happening, knows that it will pass, and knows that as long as he keeps taking his medication, the panic attacks will be few and far between.

"I look at it like somebody who needs insulin every day," he says. "I mean, it's not perfect, but nothing's perfect. I have a few side effects, like being a little sleepy sometimes during the day or awake at night, but I'll take that. Believe me, I feel a *lot* better."

ANXIETY IN ALL ITS GUISES

Isaac's story illustrates many key features of anxiety disorders: the classic fear-related body sensations; the way symptoms can mysteriously appear; the common coexistence of depression and anxiety; the difficulty of finding effective treatment without the help of a knowledgeable doctor; and the confusion and frustration caused by most people's inability to understand the condition. Isaac suffered from a specific type of anxiety: panic disorder. But the nature of his struggles and the possibility for successful treatment apply to all of the anxiety disorders we'll consider here.

Afflicting roughly 19 million people, anxiety disorders are the most common mental ills in America today.[1] Nearly everyone knows somebody with an anxiety disorder — though, of course, many people hide the condition, so even close friends or relatives may not be aware of it. About 30 percent of women and 19 percent of men in the United States will be affected by an anxiety disorder at some time in their lives.[2]

The various types of anxiety appear to share some common biology, but they affect different types of people and respond differently to medications and psychotherapy. We will cover the four most common: social anxiety disorder, posttraumatic stress disorder, generalized anxiety disorder, and panic disorder. People dealing with these illnesses invariably suffer a set of common symptoms — though what triggers them may vary widely. These symptoms may include the following:

- Feelings of intense fear, dread, or terror
- Racing or pounding heart
- Dry mouth or difficulty swallowing
- Rapid, shallow breathing
- Muscle tension

- Dizziness or vertigo
- Numbness or tingling in hands, feet, or mouth
- Trembling
- Hot or cold flashes
- A sense of depersonalization or separateness from one's body during or after an attack
- Fear of "going crazy" or losing self-control

Of course, almost everyone experiences some of these conditions at some point in their lives. That's because, as we noted in Chapter 1, anxiety itself is not a disorder — it's a valuable physical response honed by millions of years of natural selection to prepare us for a potential threat. Faced with an exam, a work deadline, or a performance, mild anxiety can impel us to study, work hard, or practice so that we can achieve our goals. If a tornado, a mugger, or a rattlesnake appears, anxiety can be a lifesaver. A normal person's feelings in these situations are no different from the anxiety that someone with an anxiety disorder feels. What makes the disorder distinct is not the quality of the anxiety but the frequency of anxiety attacks, the appropriateness of the anxiety in a given situation, and the degree to which the anxiety interferes with life.

In Isaac's case, for instance, the attacks were unrelated to actual danger, they were frequent, and they eventually interfered significantly with his life. Clearly Isaac's inborn anxiety circuits were not working as nature designed them.

NATURE'S PLAN

We'll illustrate nature's plan for the brain's anxiety circuitry by telling a story and then reviewing it in slow motion to explore what is going on "behind the scenes" in brain and body. First, the scene: You are walking alone at night along a dimly lit sidewalk. In the distance two men wearing dark clothes cross the street and walk toward you. Before you have actually thought about it, your heart starts to pound, your palms go sweaty, and you begin to breathe more rapidly. You continue to walk, but you are now alert, eyes darting first to the men, to assess their threat potential, and then in other directions, to assess possible avenues of escape. Your mind races — are you carrying much money? Would anyone hear you if you shouted for help? Should you run now and risk looking foolish or wait a few seconds to decide? You slow down a bit to give yourself some extra time. In a moment the men will be near enough that you'll be able to see their faces clearly . . . but that could be too late. Your heart now thuds in your chest, and you feel tingly from adrenaline.

Then one of the men laughs. They are talking to each other, not looking directly at you. Again, even before you think rationally about it, your heart rate begins to slow. The next second the men sweep past you, but it is fifteen minutes before your body feels normal again. A week later you can still recall the incident vividly.

Now let's run this scenario again in slow motion, using a magic camera that can peer inside your head, so that we can observe your complicated anxiety machinery in action.

First, your eyes capture images of the two men crossing the street. Your retinas convert the images to electrical impulses that surge along two cablelike nerve fibers leading from the back of each eyeball to the back of the brain, where the image-processing circuitry is located. Before those signals get there, however, they pass through a primitive, first-pass filter deep in the brain that is primed to detect potential threats. Some of this programming is "hard-wired" by genes to respond to threats that our species has faced for eons. Most of the programming in this brain region, however, is learned as we go about our lives — for instance, by watching movies involving muggings or, worse, by an actual mugging.

This first-pass filter is called the visual thalamus, and most of the time it passively relays visual signals streaming in from the eyes. But if the signals even vaguely match an image stored in memory, the visual thalamus responds within milliseconds with a volley of electrical signals to twin brain structures called the amygdalas. (For simplicity we'll watch just one amygdala in action.)

The amygdala is sometimes called the brain's "fear center" because it becomes activated in response to real or perceived danger. The amygdala receives messages from all the senses as well as from other parts of the brain, such as memory centers and the so-called executive areas involved with reason, analysis, and planning: the medial prefrontal cortex, orbital frontal cortex, and anterior cingulate.

Jolted now by the visual thalamus, the amygdala responds, sending signals in many directions. It fires up a nearby region called the hippocam-

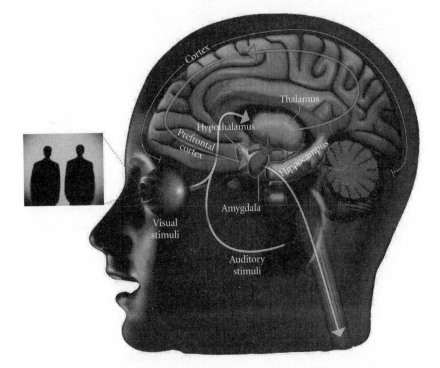

FIGURE 4. *The basic anxiety circuitry of the brain.* Sensory images of two men coming toward a person pass through the eyes, ears, and possibly other sensory organs into the thalamus. The thalamus both signals the amygdala and hypothalamus and passes the information to the cortex for processing. Stimulation of the cortex brings a perceived threat to awareness and allows for analysis and response. If stimulatory signals are too vigorous or are triggered inappropriately, or if the capacity of the cortex to override these signals is impaired, an anxiety disorder may result. *Time*, June 10, 2002, 50–51. Copyright 2002, Time Inc. Reprinted with modifications by permission.

pus, a key part of the memory system. This immediate "priming" of memory ensures that you will remember the context in which fear arose, the better to avoid such a situation in the future. The amygdala also stimulates the hypothalamus, a vital link between brain and body. The hypothalamus fires off neural messages of its own and also secretes hormones that act on other parts of the brain and body. The immediate nerve signal travels to the adrenal glands on top of the kidneys. These glands respond by dumping adrenaline into the blood, which, within seconds, speeds heart rate, releases sugar into the blood, constricts blood vessels in the extremities, shuts down digestion, and prepares for either fight or flight. At the same time the hypothalamus squirts out a hormone with the tongue-twisting name of cortico-tropin-releasing hormone (CRH for short). This hormone's target is just next door: the pituitary gland, a.k.a the body's "master gland" because it se-cretes so many important hormones.

Bathed in CRH, the pituitary gland releases its own hormone, which reaches the adrenal glands within seconds and releases cortisol, a hormone that amplifies and sustains the action of the previously released adrenaline. In the background of these various neural alert systems is the neurotrans-mitter norepinephrine, the proper levels of which are needed for a well-bal-anced fear response.

This is why your heart is pounding and you feel tingly and suddenly alert. Your body has automatically shifted to high alert even as your mind is still catching up.

The original visual image of the two men, remember, triggered the thalamus and amygdala to launch the alert, but those images were also passed on to the visual center at the back of the head. The processed images then travel to the cortex, which is the largest part of the brain. A portion of the cortex called the prefrontal cortex is the part that thinks, reasons, inter-prets, invents, and perceives itself. In short, "you" reside in your prefrontal cortex. The prefrontal cortex is much more sophisticated than the amyg-dala — it can tap your vast array of memories and take into account ab-stract ideas such as a concern for looking foolish. It can weigh and sift evi-dence from all the senses to come up with a probability of risk. But the cost of this sophistication is time. Even with your mind racing, you still haven't decided what to do.

Meanwhile, your body is panicking, and as the prefrontal cortex real-izes this fact, new nerve signals travel from the cortex back to the amygdala, strengthening its firing and amplifying the state of alert. You have almost been brought to a standstill by your fear when you hear the man laugh. The sound is interpreted by the prefrontal cortex as a sign of safety. In the next instant the men pass, and the threat is gone.

Now a host of vitally important processes begins, designed to shut down the state of alert and return body and mind to normal physiological levels. As helpful as adrenaline and cortisol are in the short term, their pres-ence hurts the body over the long term. The physiological responses they trigger — such as dampening the immune system, raising blood pressure, and raising blood sugar — are harmful if sustained.

In a resilient individual, many factors work to rapidly bring the body

back to normal. The prefrontal cortex, for instance, sends dampening signals to the amygdala. Meanwhile, receptors for cortisol in the amygdala,
hypothalamus, and pituitary detect the unusually high levels of that hormone and shut down the production of CRH, which, in turn, turns off the
cortisol "spigot."

Anxiety disorders arise if either the initial alarm system is hypersensitive or overreactive or if the systems for extinguishing the alarm are not
strong enough. Both the "on" and "off" systems are complex and involve
neurotransmitters such as norepinephrine, hormones such as adrenaline
and cortisol, memory and "executive functioning" brain regions, and many
other factors and mechanisms, any one of which can malfunction.

The Roots of Anxiety

Despite the brain's complexity, great progress has been made in the past
decade in unraveling the neurobiology of anxiety. This new understanding
promises more specific, effective, and rationally prescribed treatments for
anxiety in the future.

Of course, the biology of anxiety — the neurotransmitters, hormones,
and circuits — is inextricably entwined with the psychology of anxiety —
one's experiences, memories, conditioning, and feelings. Old distinctions
between "nature" (one's genes and biology) and "nurture" (one's upbringing and subsequent psychology) have faded with the recognition that these
forces are almost always simultaneously working to shape who we are at
any given moment. For instance, if a child with a genetic predisposition to
anxiety is born into a crisis-ridden family, the interaction of genes and environment will raise the child's risk for an anxiety disorder. On the other
hand, if the same child is born into a stable family, the environment will
help buffer the effects of genes, lowering the risk of a later disorder.

Genes

No single "anxiety gene" exists, unlike the single genetic malfunctions at
the root of sickle-cell anemia, Huntington disease, or other rare conditions.
But genes certainly set the stage for anxiety. Family studies show that the
more closely related a person is to an anxious relative (that is, the more
genes shared with him or her), the higher the individual's chances of hav-

ing a disorder as well. Three major studies found that if a parent or a sibling has panic disorder, a person's risk of having it is roughly 15 percent, compared to the general risk of about 4 percent.[3] An intriguing 2003 study, by Ken Kendler and his colleagues at the Virginia Institute for Psychiatric and Behavioral Genetics, found that genes play a significant role in the acquisition and extinction of the fear response.[4] Specifically, the fear responses of pairs of identical and fraternal twins were studied, and the results show that the heritability of similar fear responses is about 40 percent.

Studies of panic disorder among identical twins who were reared in different homes show that if one twin has panic disorder, the other twin has roughly a 50 percent chance of also having the disorder. Progress has been made in finding the relevant genes. Steven Hamilton and his colleagues at Columbia University reported in 2003 that genes on chromosomes 13q and 22 were significantly linked to panic disorder.[5] Some other recent work illuminates a genetic basis for the observation that many people prone to panic attacks are also very sensitive to stimulants such as caffeine. Karen Alsene and her colleagues at the University of Chicago found a specific genetic alteration that predisposed those with the alteration to become anxious in response to caffeine.[6]

Such research clearly suggests the likelihood that many genes and gene variations participate in setting a biological vulnerability to anxiety disorders, each one contributing only slightly to an overall tendency. But the work also proves that genes are not destiny. Even if you share all your genes with somebody (an identical twin), you still have only a fifty-fifty chance of sharing an anxiety disorder, and none of the gene studies find a specific alteration in all the people studied. As with most other medical disorders, the influence of genes is greatly affected by other factors.

Upbringing

The family in which a person grows up can increase or decrease his or her risk for a wide range of mental illnesses, including anxiety disorders. Generally speaking, stress, poverty, psychological difficulties, violence, neglect, or abuse in a family increases risk, while stability, emotional health, and loving support lower that risk.[7] Most families, of course, fall somewhere in the middle, with some degree of dysfunction and distress coexisting with some degree of stability and love. Objectively evaluating where on this hypothetical scale a family falls can be difficult because people know their families intimately but know other families only from a distance — and families typically try to hide their dysfunction. It may seem, in other words, that one's family is much more "crazy" and dysfunctional than normal when, in fact, it falls squarely in the normal range.

For instance, experiencing a divorce as a child is always a difficult and painful event, but the mere fact of a divorce in your background does not mean you come from a dysfunctional family or that you are subsequently at risk. What matters is not the divorce but the circumstances surrounding it, the way the divorce was handled, and whether it increased or decreased stress, stability, and opportunities for emotional attachment.

When evaluating upbringing as a possible contributing cause of an anxiety disorder, look for two factors: family stress (particularly during infancy and childhood) and the emotional attachment between children and the parents (primarily, but not necessarily, the mother).

Stress on a child can come from many sources, including the following:

- Psychiatric illness of a parent
- Extreme poverty
- Physical, emotional, or sexual abuse
- Neglect
- Severe, repeated parental conflict
- Death of a parent
- Loss of contact with one or both parents through abandonment, divorce, imprisonment, or state-imposed custody
- Living in a high-crime, high-violence neighborhood
- Substance abuse or addiction in one or both parents
- Chronic medical illness (such as that requiring a long stay in a pediatric intensive care unit, repeated hospitalization, and so on)

Each of these stressors involves both psychological and physiological dynamics. Research described in 2002 in the journal *Biological Psychiatry*, for instance, shows that sustained high levels of stress in the first four and a half years of a child's life strongly correlate with sustained higher-than-normal levels of the adrenal stress hormone cortisol in the child.[8] Children with raised cortisol levels had more emotional and behavioral difficulties when they entered school. In this study new mothers were regularly screened in the first year of their child's life for depression, anger, parenting stress, responsibility for filling multiple roles, and financial stress. When the mothers and their children were measured at the end of the period, the children of the mothers who were in the highest-stress group, both in infancy and at the study's conclusion, were the ones with significantly raised cortisol levels. The study also contained some good news. Children whose mothers were stressed during infancy but not later had normal cortisol levels, suggesting that if the stress ends, cortisol levels can return to normal. Likewise, the children whose mothers were stressed only at the end of the study also had normal cortisol levels, implying that experiencing an infancy without stress conferred some resilience when facing later stress.

This study is just one of many painting similar pictures. Vulnerability to anxiety (and depression as well) is increased by high stress during childhood and is decreased by strong emotional attachments during childhood.[9] Physiological stress to the fetus during pregnancy likely has a similar deleterious effect. A great deal of animal research shows that both prenatal and early-life stress profoundly alters a variety of neurotransmitter and hormone systems in ways that resemble the profiles of anxious or depressed humans.[10] Again, such research doesn't mean people can't recover from early stress or trauma — it just illustrates the power of one's environment to sculpt both psychology and neurology.

LIFE TRIGGERS

If genes and upbringing load the anxiety-disorder gun, a specific life event can sometimes pull the trigger and produce an actual anxiety or panic attack. Even when a first attack seems to come out of nowhere, life triggers may be at work — they may simply not be recognized for what they are. But just as often the corrosive effects of a genetic vulnerability and a stressful upbringing prime the anxiety circuits to overreact, react at inappropriate times, or fail to restore equilibrium following trauma.

Here, listed in roughly the order of their potential significance, are the life events most likely to trigger an anxiety disorder:

- Rape
- Physical assault
- Combat

- Sudden death of a loved one
- Accidents
- Natural disaster
- Witnessing a death or injury
- Medications
- Being in an enclosed space without easy exit
- Onset of a new medical illness
- Terrorist attacks

Most people who experience one of these events will not succumb to an anxiety disorder because their inborn anxiety machinery, their social support system, and their level of psychological resilience allow them to absorb the blow and recover. But for those vulnerable by virtue of their genes, early life experiences, or upbringing, such events can be devastating.

One trigger listed here deserves elaboration: medications. Many drugs — both therapeutic and recreational — can trigger anxiety symptoms or even full-blown panic attacks in vulnerable individuals. Many over-the-counter decongestants, sleep medications, cough suppressants, and allergy medications contain stimulating compounds that can exacerbate anxiety symptoms. Caffeine, the world's most frequently consumed stimulant, can also worsen anxiety. Eliminating caffeine from the diet often reduces anxiety symptoms dramatically. (For a more complete list of drugs that can cause or worsen anxiety, see Appendix III.)

These triggers combine with genes and upbringing in many complex ways, which is one reason for the range of anxiety disorders. We'll now look more closely at the four main types, discussed in order of their prevalence in the U.S. population.

SOCIAL ANXIETY DISORDER

Ricky Williams had made it.[11] After winning the Heisman Trophy while at the University of Texas in 1999, the New Orleans Saints gave up all of their draft picks for him, a "first" in NFL history. He was famous, wealthy, and talented. Unfortunately, he also suffered from a debilitating shyness that became acute when the pressure and fame increased.

"I've always been shy, but in New Orleans there were times my shyness would cause me actual physical pain," he says. "I'd get so claustrophobic around people that I'd bend over from the sickness in my stomach. That's not a good way to be when you're famous."

Ricky took to wearing his football helmet during television interviews — a habit that led to a reputation for being "weird" and "standoffish."

"The helmet created distance," he says, "a shield between my insecurities and the cameras and lights. But in trying to push attention away, I ended up attracting more. A lot of things in New Orleans backfired on me that way."

Ricky missed four games his rookie year because of elbow and ankle injuries. In his second season he rushed for one thousand yards but played only the first ten games because he broke an ankle. By season's end he felt awful.

"Here I was, a young man, a millionaire, sitting at home not wanting to leave, and my relationships with my mom, my sisters, and my daughter were all miserable," he says.

On the advice of a friend Ricky sought professional help in 2001 and was quickly diagnosed with social anxiety disorder. He began taking an antidepressant, which is a common treatment, as well as attending regular therapy sessions. In 2002 he was traded to the Miami Dolphins, and he played all season and became the NFL's leading rusher. He no longer wears a helmet during interviews and credits his treatment with a profound change in his attitude and outlook.

"I tell people I was a caterpillar locked in a cocoon, but now I feel like I finally have my wings," he says.

Social anxiety disorder has been called the "neglected" anxiety disorder because, despite its prevalence, the medical and mental health communities have not given it much attention until recently. Its symptoms reflect the discomfort and hesitancy many "normal" people feel when faced with public speaking, performing, or functioning in social settings with unfamiliar people. But these feelings are greatly exaggerated in those with social anxiety disorder, and they lead to disruption and dysfunction in life. Symptoms include the following when present in the context of a social setting: heart palpitations, tremors, sweating, diarrhea, confusion, intense fear of embarrassment, or avoidance of social situations that disrupts one's life.

People with social anxiety disorder typically don't have shortness of breath or think they are going to die (unlike those with panic disorder). They also don't have attacks in the middle of the night or "out of nowhere," as do those with panic disorder. This supports the idea that it is a distinct dysfunction — though the exact malfunction in the relevant brain circuitry has not yet been found.

Social anxiety disorder affects about 5 million adult Americans.[12] Women are somewhat more vulnerable — roughly 16 percent of women and 11 percent of men are afflicted, making it the most common anxiety disorder. It usually begins in childhood or early adolescence. Research also shows that people with social anxiety disorder are at a higher risk for substance abuse problems because they often try to self-medicate with alcohol or other drugs.[13]

Two subtypes of the disorder exist: generalized social anxiety, marked by fear of a wide range of social situations and contacts, and nongeneralized social anxiety, which arises in only one or two specific situations, such as stage performances.[14] Generalized social anxiety tends to compromise one's quality of life more seriously than does the more specific type. People with both types tend to be extremely sensitive to how other people perceive them. They fear their mind will "go blank" if they speak as the center of attention, that they'll say foolish things if asked to speak, or that they will tremble and shake so much that their condition will be obvious to everyone.

Much research is now under way to pin down the psychological and biological foundations of social anxiety disorder. Genes appear to play a role by setting a general tendency toward fearfulness — a trait labeled "behavioral inhibition" by the Harvard psychologist Jerome Kagan. Children identified as being inhibited at age two are twice as likely as uninhibited peers to experience social anxiety disorder in adolescence. Malfunctions or imbalances in some of the brain's key neurotransmitter systems, particularly those involving serotonin and norepinephrine, have also been implicated. Some recent studies also show a variety of potentially important dysfunctions in the neurotransmitter dopamine, which, among other things, affects how extraverted and outwardly directed a person feels. Dopamine, however, is just one player in a very complicated neurobiological drama. Irregularities in other neurotransmitter systems or brain circuits are also undoubtedly involved.

Like other psychological illnesses, social anxiety disorder may result from a progressive destabilization of brain function that begins with relatively small perturbations in the norepinephrine and serotonin systems.

These initially small changes may lead to excessive release of hormones such as corticotropin-releasing hormone, which, in turn, amplify the initially small changes in norepinephrine and serotonin. Several negative feedback loops can be generated, all of which can be affected by one's surroundings.

Research into the biology and anatomy of social behavior is being actively pursued, and early results are intriguing. For example, Murray Stein and his colleagues at the University of California–San Diego showed that when people with social anxiety disorder are shown images of contemptuous or angry faces, their amygdala and other related brain structures are significantly more active than those of normal subjects.[15] These results support work in animal research, suggesting a pivotal role for the amygdala in both the fear response and human social behavior.

Because social anxiety disorder is linked to both biology and psychology, both medications and psychotherapy can effectively relieve symptoms. (See Chapter 5 for more details.) Nobody knows how many people fail to get help for this disorder, but we suspect it is a large proportion of the affected population. Like Ricky Williams, many people don't know they have a well-studied, clinically distinct disorder with clear biological roots. That's a shame because this particular disorder can be very successfully treated these days.

POSTTRAUMATIC STRESS DISORDER (PTSD)

Many people think of war veterans when they hear the phrase "posttraumatic stress disorder," but PTSD afflicts far more people than that. In fact, PTSD is now recognized as the second most common anxiety disorder, and combat vets make up only a small proportion of the total PTSD population, which is estimated to be about 5 million adults and an unestimated number of children.[16]

Here, in her own words, is the brief story of P. K. Philips, which vividly illustrates some common themes of this disorder:

> In my case PTSD was triggered by several traumas, including a childhood laced with physical, mental, and sexual abuse, and later, by an attack at knifepoint, which left me thinking I would die. I would never be the same after that attack. For me there was no safe place in the world,

not even my home. I went to the police and filed a report. Rape counselors came to see me while I was in the hospital, but I declined their help, convinced that I didn't need it. This would be the most damaging decision of my life.

For months after the attack, I couldn't close my eyes without envisioning the face of my attacker. I suffered horrific flashbacks and nightmares. For four years after the attack I was unable to sleep alone in my house. I obsessively checked windows, doors, and locks. By age seventeen, I suffered my first panic attack. The attacks continued, and I soon became unable to leave my apartment for weeks at a time, ending my modeling career abruptly. This just became a way of life. Years passed during which I had few or no symptoms at all, and I led what I thought was a fairly normal life, just thinking I had a "panic problem."

Four years ago another traumatic event retriggered the PTSD. It was as if all the years had evaporated, and I was back in the place of my attack, only now I had uncontrollable thoughts of someone entering my house and harming my daughter. I saw violent images every time I closed my eyes. I lost all ability to concentrate or even complete simple tasks. Normally social, I stopped trying to make friends or get involved in my community. I often felt disoriented, forgetting where, or who, I was — which was terrifying. I would panic on the freeway and became unable to drive, again ending my career. I felt like I had completely lost my mind. For a time, I managed to keep it together on the outside, but then I became unable to leave my house again.

Around this time I was diagnosed with PTSD. I cannot express the enormous relief I felt when I discovered my condition was real and treatable. I felt safe for the first time in thirty-two years. I began taking medication, which in combination with behavioral therapy, marked the turning point in regaining control of my life. I completed an intensive three weeks of prolonged exposure therapy, which finally got me out of my house and slowly back into a full life. I'm working again and rebuilding a satisfying career as an artist. I am enjoying my life — the world is new to me and not limited by the restrictive vision of anxiety. It amazes me to think back to what my life was like only a year ago and to realize just how far I've come.

As P.K.'s story shows, PTSD can develop after exposure to a terrifying event or ordeal in which grave physical harm occurred or was threatened.

Traumatic events that involve deliberate assault by another person, such as a mugging or a rape, are particularly powerful triggers, as is abuse or assault by someone with whom one has an emotional or dependent relationship. Other types of trauma can induce PTSD as well, such as witnessing violence, death, or injury; military combat; natural or human-caused disasters; and being the object of terrorism.

Sometimes symptoms appear immediately, but they may be delayed for months or years. The diagnosis of PTSD requires that at least one of the following symptoms be present for at least one month in the context of an experienced traumatic event:

- Repeated reexperiencing of the ordeal in the form of flashbacks, memories, nightmares, or frightening thoughts, especially with exposure to events or objects reminiscent of the original trauma
- Emotional numbness
- Sleep disturbances
- Depression
- Anxiety and irritability
- Feelings of intense guilt
- Headaches, gastrointestinal complaints, immune system problems, dizziness, or chest pain

As with anxiety disorders in general, PTSD may arise from malfunctions in either (or both) of two general brain systems: the alarm system (also called the fear-conditioning system) and the extinction systems that bring body and mind back to normal after a frightening or stressful experience. As noted earlier, many hormones and neurotransmitters are involved, as are several brain regions, particularly those involved with memory formation.

Even very resilient people will suffer some of the listed symptoms when exposed to a traumatic experience. But with healthy anxiety and extinction systems, these symptoms typically abate over the course of days or, at most, a few weeks, the physical symptoms disappear, and the person is able to function socially and vocationally. At a psychological level, the trauma becomes integrated and accepted into the larger life context and therefore does not become an isolated, unacknowledged mental "cancer." By talking with others, working to accept the consequences of the trauma, and taking steps to deal with those consequences, a resilient individual can come to terms with even horrific trauma and continue functioning. (Children, of course, often do not have the psychological resources or maturity to deal effectively with trauma, and for them, a great deal of care and support must be provided. For more detail, see Chapter 12.)

But if the extinction systems are compromised, memories will become intrusive and uncontrollable, accompanied by surges of fear or terror created by anxiety mechanisms pitched at high alert despite the absence of a real threat. One of the brain structures involved in the extinction of conditioned responses and memory storage is the hippocampus, and some studies have found that the size of the hippocampus is reduced in many people with PTSD.[17] It's not yet clear whether this size reduction is caused by the hormone surges that occur during trauma or whether the hippocampus in such people is smaller from birth, leaving them more vulnerable to PTSD.

Memories, even traumatic ones, are not as fixed as was once thought. Recent research suggests that when a memory is retrieved from long-term storage and held in one's attention, it becomes part of one's present intellectual and emotional reality. As such, new connections can be made with the memories — connections that can serve to stabilize and minimize the associated bodily responses. Active memories can then be reconsolidated and stored in long-term memory, with new, and potentially more resilient, connections. For example, a frightening childhood memory involving a feeling of abandonment can be recalled in a safe and secure environment and linked to the less emotionally vulnerable understandings and perspective of adulthood.

At a biological level, too, memories brought into current awareness can be manipulated in some ways. Preclinical studies have shown that introducing certain chemical compounds when a memory is being retrieved can reduce the strength of the original traumatic memory.[18] The same phenomenon has been demonstrated with memory-dampening drugs administered after a traumatic event. Both of these findings promise better ways to deal with acute trauma and to treat those still suffering from past trauma.

Other biological irregularities may be involved in PTSD, such as elevated levels of corticotropin-releasing hormone or extrasensitivity in the release and functioning of the neurotransmitter norepinephrine. Scott Rauch and colleagues at Harvard Medical School found in 2003 that some specific brain structures known to be involved in PTSD, such as the anterior cingulate, were smaller in a group of women with PTSD, compared with the brain structures of a control group, further illustrating the tangled biological roots of this disorder.[19]

Complicating the diagnosis and treatment of PTSD is the fact that depression, substance abuse, alcoholism, and other anxiety disorders commonly occur at the same time as PTSD. Sometimes a problem, such as alcoholism, begins as a response to the PTSD but then acquires a life of its own and may become an even greater source of dysfunction than the PTSD. Treating the PTSD can sometimes have a positive impact on co-occurring problems, but it is equally likely that the co-occurring problems must be effectively treated before progress can be made on the PTSD.

Fortunately, a combination of psychotherapy and medications has been shown to be relatively effective in treating most cases of PTSD, which, when left untreated, can be exceptionally disabling.

GENERALIZED ANXIETY DISORDER (GAD)

If you met Kathy (a pseudonym) in her professional life as a physician's assistant, you would see a woman with apparent confidence, a sense of humor, energy, and compassion for her patients and colleagues. You would not see the grinding worry that gnaws at her almost every day. You would not see the pain caused by "flashes" of horrible accidents happening to her children, which sometimes appear as unbidden visions. You wouldn't see the two glasses of wine at the end of the day that calm her nerves. And you wouldn't see the immense emotional energy required to subdue the fears and the worry so that she can function at work and at home.

Kathy lives in the gray zone between normalcy and dysfunction. Some days she feels truly disabled — so consumed with tension, worry, and "nerves" that she feels nauseated, forgetful, and unfocused. Some days she is fine — competent, secure, and happy. Most days are somewhere in between — she functions, but always with a gnawing, low-grade worry — a kind of emotional static that, she says, keeps her from being the person she really wants to be.

All her life she has fought to be calmer, more relaxed, less keyed up. She knows that meditating and exercise help, but often she's either too tired or just too wound up for that. She knows caffeine makes the anxiety worse, but without it she feels unbearably tired. An intelligent woman with years of therapy under her belt, she knows, too, that her excessive worry is related to both the genes and the psychology she got from her mother, who was emotionally distant, hypercritical, and herself prone to exaggerated and irrational fears.

Still, Kathy feels powerless against the worry most of the time and cherishes the moments — usually on weekends or a vacation — when she is distracted or relaxed and the anxiety recedes.

Kathy has generalized anxiety disorder, a subtle, long-term emotional malfunction that erodes quality of life by making it impossible to relax. Generalized anxiety disorder (GAD) afflicts millions of people in the United States — roughly 4 percent of the population.[20] The most prominent features of the disorder are excessive thinking and dwelling on the "what ifs" in life. If a loved one is ten minutes late, for instance, someone with generalized anxiety fears the worst. Vivid scenarios of accidents or death rush through the mind, triggering a flood of fear, anxiety, and adrenaline-linked physical effects. Elements of social anxiety disorder and/or panic may sometimes be present, such as high levels of self-consciousness in some situations, but no single "target" for worry exists. Unlike the symptoms of panic disorder or social anxiety disorder, the worry associated with GAD can attach itself to anything. People with GAD often have an exaggerated startle reflex — sudden noises make them jump — and they sometimes seem to be in constant motion.

The formal definition of GAD is a state of excessive worry and anxiety that is difficult or impossible to control during at least half the days of a six-month period. In addition, an affected person experiences at least three of the following symptoms regularly during the same period: restlessness, muscle tension, fatigue, irritability, sleep disturbances, or difficulty concentrating.

People with GAD suffer with difficult symptoms but typically are not crippled by them, as are those with other types of anxiety or major depression. Often, like Kathy, they are successful in their careers and relationships. But the suffering is real, and those with GAD are at higher risk for other disorders. By one estimate, nine of every ten people with chronic GAD have experienced another psychiatric disorder such as major depression, dysthymia (a low-grade depression), a phobia, or substance abuse.[21]

GAD is the least studied of the anxiety disorders, in part because it was not recognized as a distinct clinical entity until 1980. It is very likely that people with GAD have an underlying malfunction or hypersensitivity of the inborn anxiety circuits, but the exact malfunction remains unclear. Whatever the biological roots, the resulting interaction with the people and circumstances of life can result in a spectrum of maladaptive psychological responses such as the feeling of being "nervous," "a worrier," or "foolish." Fortunately, both psychotherapeutic and pharmacological treatments for GAD have proved highly effective. (Chapter 5 describes treatment options.)

PANIC DISORDER

As illustrated by Isaac's story at the beginning of this chapter, panic disorder is characterized by unexpected and repeated attacks of intense fear accompanied by physical symptoms, which may include chest pain, heart palpitations, shortness of breath, dizziness or lightheadedness, tingling, chills or blushing, or hot flashes. These sensations can resemble symptoms of a heart attack, and, as a result, the diagnosis of panic disorder is often not made until extensive and costly medical procedures fail to provide a correct diagnosis or relief.

Panic attacks usually begin abruptly and build to maximum intensity within fifteen minutes. Most people report a fear of dying, "going crazy," or losing control of their emotions or behavior. Attacks generally provoke a strong urge to escape or flee the place where they began. They rarely last longer than thirty minutes.

Not everyone who has a panic attack has panic disorder, however. Roughly one of every ten adults will have an isolated panic attack in any given year.[22] In addition, panic attacks may be experienced by those with another, more primary psychological condition, such as social anxiety disorder, generalized anxiety disorder, or major depression.

Panic disorder is diagnosed only if a person has experienced at least two panic attacks and changes his or her behavior to avoid or minimize such attacks or develops persistent worry about having further attacks. Whereas the number and severity of the attacks vary widely, the related concern and avoidance behavior are common and similar among sufferers. As with other anxiety disorders, people with panic disorder often have other conditions such as depression (estimated to co-occur in 50 to 65 percent of patients) and substance abuse disorders. Panic disorder afflicts about 2.5 million American adults between ages eighteen and fifty-four, and it is about twice as common among women as men.[23]

Isaac's case was also typical in that the panic attacks eventually involved acute agoraphobia as well. The term *agoraphobia* comes from the Greek word for "open marketplace" (*agora*), but this condition is more complicated than a simple fear of open spaces. People with agoraphobia typically have a severe and pervasive anxiety about being in situations from which escape might be difficult, such as being on bridges, traveling in a car, bus, or airplane, or being in a crowded area. In this sense it shares some features of claustrophobia, the fear of being in a confined space.

Although panic attacks may begin as a purely biological malfunction, a powerful learned component quickly sets in. As panic attacks become more frequent, a person often begins to avoid situations in which he or she fears another attack may occur or help would not be immediately available. This avoidance may eventually develop into an inability to go beyond known and safe surroundings, such as a house or apartment, because of intense fear and anxiety.

The neurobiology of panic disorder is beginning to come to light. Like other mental afflictions, it points to a complicated machinery that can go awry in many ways, each way leading to the same experience of panic. For example, studies to date have found the following conditions in patients with panic disorder:

- Alterations in levels of the neurotransmitter norepinephrine
- Reduced numbers of receptors to which norepinephrine and serotonin attach themselves
- Oversensitivity of the amygdala
- Blunted responsiveness in the HPA axis
- Enhanced sensitivity to caffeine
- Enhanced activity of other important brain compounds called neuropeptides[24]

Malfunctions in any of these systems might predispose a person to panic by making the alarm system go off too easily or too often or by making it more difficult to dampen an alarm signal once it happens.

The observation that nearly everyone with panic disorder experiences shortness of breath or a feeling of suffocation during an attack points to another type of biological disorder that may play a role. The brain contains a small cluster of cells that constantly monitors the level of the waste gas carbon dioxide (CO_2) in the blood. When CO_2 levels rise, for instance, because of exercise, these cells detect the change and tell the lungs and heart to work faster, which brings the levels back down. Studies have shown that some people with panic disorder have a hypersensitive respiratory control system, which sends false signals of suffocation that in turn cause breathlessness and intense feelings of fear, dread, and danger.[25]

Genes undoubtedly play a role in panic disorder, though the task of pinpointing the likely genetic culprits is just beginning. Researchers at the University of Seoul, South Korea, for example, found much higher rates of abnormal versions of a gene related to the metabolism of adrenaline among a set of fifty-one patients with panic disorder.[26] Other genetic irregularities probably lie at the root of the neurotransmitter and hormonal variations described in this chapter.

The bottom line is that panic disorder — like most diseases — tends to run in families and does not result from "weak character" or a "flawed personality." What is now considered a single psychological disorder — panic — will most likely prove to be a cluster of underlying biological disorders, all of which interact with a person's upbringing and life experiences to influence overall vulnerability to panic disorder. Recognizing this biological component can be a tremendous relief to people with panic disorder because the symptoms are so confusing and debilitating. Fortunately, as with the other anxiety disorders, effective treatments are now available, as we will discuss in the next chapter.

5

FINDING OPTIMAL RELIEF
FROM ANXIETY DISORDERS

Happy is the man who has broken the chains that hurt the mind, and
has given up worrying, once and for all.

— OVID

ALMOST EVERYONE with an anxiety disorder can be helped, and most
people can be helped so much that their symptoms can be eliminated. We
would like to say that most people can be "cured," but that is not generally
the case with anxiety disorders (or depression). As with diabetes or familial
high cholesterol, the biological dysfunctions usually involved with anxiety
disorders do not disappear even when the symptoms of the dysfunction are
under control. The only caveat related to our positive attitude is that successful treatment usually requires commitment, patience, and no small
amount of hard work on the part of the patient.

Far too many people fail to get the relief they desire and deserve. They
and their medical practitioner may mistake a partial improvement for the
optimal improvement possible, or they may not work long enough to find
the best medication and the best dose for optimal effect. Patients and physicians also sometimes rely exclusively on a medication without addressing
the psychological dimensions of a disorder.

This chapter explains how to wring the maximum benefit from the
many treatments now available for anxiety disorders. Remember that, in
the end, success will depend on the patient's tenacity as well as the skill and
patience of the clinician.

Treatments for anxiety disorders fall into two basic groups: medications and psychotherapy. (A variety of complementary therapies may
enhance these basic approaches; these are reviewed and discussed in Appendix I.)

Many people see the two types of treatment, medications and psychotherapy, as distinct or even as antagonistic to each other. This is both un-

true and unhelpful. Medications work on the brain, and by modifying or correcting the mechanisms underlying an anxiety disorder, they reduce or eliminate fearfulness, nervousness, and other worrisome ways of thinking and feeling. In short, medications work directly on the brain and indirectly on the mind. Psychotherapies work the opposite way: directly on the mind and indirectly on the brain. Remember that learning changes the brain; hence, when a person talks with a therapist, reflects on a situation, listens to others, or learns about a condition, he or she is sculpting the brain's "wiring." Such learning may bring new ways to view the disorder itself, a greater ability to accept and integrate painful past experiences, or more positive ways to think about life circumstances.

We want to press this point. In this era, insight and learning can be easily overshadowed by medications. After all, swallowing a pill is easy, while facing fears, acknowledging past denial, understanding complicated family dynamics, and dealing with other people can be difficult. Psychotherapy also unavoidably takes time — something in chronically short supply these days. But we urge patients to take psychotherapy seriously and engage in the work involved. Dozens of studies demonstrate that combining medication with psychotherapy produces better outcomes than either medication alone or psychotherapy alone.[1] The insight and learning that can result from good psychotherapy are invaluable and can never be put in a pill. Such knowledge can be the key to moving beyond one level of psychological fitness to greater resilience and happiness.

First Steps

The first call to make in seeking help for an anxiety disorder should be to a personal or family doctor. If one doesn't have a physician who at least has one's medical records on hand, friends or relatives should be asked for suggestions. (For more leads on finding a qualified doctor, see Appendix IV.) If one typically uses a non-Western caregiver such as an acupuncturist or naturopath, we strongly suggest seeking at least a preliminary meeting with an M.D. As helpful as alternative practices may sometimes be, we feel they are best used as a complement to, not a replacement for, contemporary medicine.

An initial meeting with a physician should involve a thorough medical history and a complete physical examination. Both can be critical for understanding a condition and directing treatment. Many medical conditions cause symptoms that mimic characteristics of anxiety disorders. Some medications produce side effects that do the same thing. Other possible causes for symptoms must be ruled out before proceeding with a specific anti-anxiety treatment. Equally important is examining one's life circumstances, cultural background, and thoughts and feelings about treatment options because these all relate to finding optimal treatment.

These days family or personal physicians commonly prescribe anti-anxiety medications. This may make sense if a physician knows the patient well and if the patient is very comfortable telling his or her doctor about embarrassing or painful life circumstances. But in our opinion, general physicians rarely have the time to determine a proper diagnosis and oversee the ongoing monitoring required to get optimal results from a medication. Family physicians are also not psychotherapists. Given the importance of psychotherapy, we suggest that everyone wondering about an anxiety disorder ask for a referral to a psychiatrist, psychologist, or other mental health worker. Appendix V explains the various types of mental health workers and how they differ from one another in training and focus.

Treating anxiety disorders with medications, psychotherapy, or both is a complicated process and requires intelligence, deep understanding of neurobiology and psychology, and a high degree of emotional intelligence (empathy, compassion, stability, insight, and a sense of humor). Regardless of title or academic degree of the chosen therapist, a therapeutic alliance with that person is what counts. One needs to feel safe, cared about, and valued for putting effort into recovery. Like any relationship, the client-therapist alliance will have ups and downs — and therapy should not be abandoned if occasional disagreement or difficulty surfaces. That said, sometimes the fit between a client and a therapist simply isn't good; at such times, another therapist should be sought. Of course, terminating a therapeutic relationship and beginning another can be tiring and frustrating, but it can make all the difference in the world.

Cabinetmaker Erik Elder's experience with the physician who first diagnosed his psychiatric problem illustrates the point. ("Erik Elder" is a pseudonym.) "When I got there," Erik says, "some young doctor walks in and says, 'I looked at your records and I'm wondering if you want to do medication and psychotherapy or whether you want to do electroshock treatment.' I said, 'Well, Doc, do you prefer an English dovetail or a French dovetail on your cabinets?' And he said, 'Well, I don't really know what you're talking about.' And I said, 'Well, how in the hell do you expect me to know what *you're* talking about? You're asking me to make that type of decision and we haven't even spent a day together?'"

Erik was so dismayed by the doctor's attitude and conduct that he simply left. Fortunately he kept looking and found a psychiatrist he respected and with whom for seven years now he has shared a strong and effective therapeutic alliance.

MEDICATIONS

Different anxiety disorders respond to different types or combinations of medications. Recall that the brain, like a car, has both "accelerator" neurotransmitters and "brake" neurotransmitters. Anxiety disorders may involve either too many "accelerator" neurotransmitters (such as norepinephrine) or too few "brake" neurotransmitters (such as gamma-aminobutyric acid, or GABA). Medications can correct such imbalances. For example, Valium (diazepam) is the best-known member of a family of medications first used decades ago to treat anxiety disorders: the benzodiazepines. All benzodiazepines have essentially the same effect on the brain, though some work faster than others or stay in the body longer than others. The medications work because their molecular shape resembles the shape of GABA. Swallowing a pill from this group floods the brain with millions of extra "brakes." Within minutes, the firing of neurons in the brain is dampened — including those causing anxiety symptoms.

Benzodiazepines Used to Treat Anxiety Disorders

TRADE NAME	GENERIC NAME
Ativan	lorazepam
Azene, Tranxene	clorazepate
Centrax	prazepam
Klonopin	clonazepam
Librium or Librax	chlordiazepoxide
Paxipam	halazepam
Serax	oxazepam
Valium	diazepam
Xanax	alprazolam

Drugs in the benzodiazepine family work rapidly and are generally effective in reducing or eliminating symptoms of anxiety and panic. They can be used occasionally on an as-needed basis or more regularly, depending on the individual's symptoms and physiological response. But these medicines also have drawbacks. Benzodiazepines don't selectively target the anxiety circuits — the entire brain is affected — which means coordination, thinking, memory, breathing, and heart rate are affected as well, especially early in the course of treatment. Benzodiazepines also induce a mild euphoria, particularly for some people, similar to the effects of alcohol. In fact, alcohol molecules act to some extent on the same GABA receptors that benzodiazepines affect. This leads to two problems: (1) benzodiazepines amplify the intoxicating effects of alcohol, making accidental overdose much easier; and (2) people vulnerable to alcoholism are also vulnerable to benzodiazepine addiction. Benzodiazepines are thus used primarily for short-term relief of symptoms or as temporary adjunct medications with newer anti-anxiety drugs. (Some people, however, can use benzodiazepines on a long-term basis without experiencing a reduction in their therapeutic effect.)

The benzodiazepines have been displaced as first-line medications for anxiety by a new class of drugs developed in the 1980s as antidepressants. Prozac (fluoxetine) was the first drug of this new type — technically called selective serotonin reuptake inhibitors, or SSRIs. Many drugs in this family have potent anti-anxiety effects as well, though some are more effective for some people than others.

The discovery that SSRIs relieve anxiety was a tremendous boon for both patients and physicians. These drugs can be safely used on a long-term basis, are not addictive, do not depress functioning in other brain areas (indeed, they sometimes improve functioning), and interact only mildly with alcohol.

SSRIs Commonly Used to Treat Anxiety Disorders

TRADE NAME	GENERIC NAME
Celexa	citalopram
Lexapro	escitalopram
Luvox	fluvoxamine
Paxil, Paxil CR (controlled release)	paroxetine
Prozac	fluoxetine
Zoloft	sertraline

A drawback of SSRIs is that therapeutic effects tend to appear only after two weeks, and the drugs can take up to eight weeks to fully kick in. This lag happens even though their actions in the brain occur rapidly. After being swallowed, these drugs typically increase levels of the neurotransmitter serotonin in the brain within about thirty minutes. The higher neuro-transmitter levels appear to cause a chain reaction elsewhere in the brain, which results in a gradual change — perhaps the growth of new connections between the brain cells themselves. In turn, these calm anxiety and lift depression.

The lag time between the start of SSRI administration and relief of anxiety symptoms can be dealt with by using a benzodiazepine in the initial weeks of treatment, so that a patient gets some immediate relief while the SSRI takes effect.[2] The benzodiazepine can be tapered off once the SSRI begins to work. This strategy takes advantage of the strengths of both classes of drugs while avoiding some of their respective drawbacks. (Because the same liver enzymes break down some benzodiazepines and some SSRIs, certain combinations of these drugs work better than others.)[3]

As good as they are, the SSRIs produce side effects for many people; some problems, such as excessive perspiration or the inability to have an orgasm, can be quite troublesome. People who are using other medications (such as some heart medications) must use SSRIs carefully because some drug combinations are hazardous. Different members of the SSRI family can affect people in different ways and produce different side effects. That's why people often try out one SSRI, and then, if they experience troublesome side effects, try others until they find one that works best for them. And, like most medications, an SSRI should not be stopped "cold turkey," but rather the dose should be tapered off over a course of weeks.

Some new medications have been introduced in recent years that are variations on the SSRI theme. Some of them raise levels of both serotonin and norepinephrine, while others work primarily on norepinephrine. These new drugs can be as good or better than the SSRIs for some patients, though some, such as Wellbutrin (bupropion), have not been shown effective in the treatment of anxiety.

Other Antidepressants Used to Treat Anxiety Disorders

TRADE NAME	GENERIC NAME
Effexor, Effexor XR (extended release)	venlafaxine
Remeron	mirtazapine
Serzone	nefazodone

Although SSRIs and other antidepressants are first-line pharmacological treatments for most types of anxiety disorders, they are not the only antidepressants that work. Two older classes of antidepressants — tricyclics and monoamine oxidase inhibitors (MAOIs) — can also alleviate anxiety symptoms. But these drugs usually produce more side effects than newer drugs do and are more hazardous in overdose; also, the old MAOIs require strict adherence to some dietary limitations. Some new types of MAOIs do not require dietary changes; these may become more commonly used in the future, but they have not yet been rigorously studied for the treatment of anxiety disorders and are not now available in the United States. Despite their limitations, however, MAOIs can be useful because they are the only medications some patients respond to.

PSYCHOTHERAPY

Overcoming anxiety and building resilience can be greatly facilitated by psychotherapy, which has been shown to be as effective as medications in relieving symptoms in some people and for some types of anxiety, though better results are usually obtained when both are combined. Psychotherapy yields insight and knowledge about a troublesome condition and how it has affected a person's life and relationships. Psychotherapy can also equip a person with new skills and coping mechanisms that can directly diminish symptoms and ward off further attacks.

Of the many types of therapy available today, studies show that cognitive-behavioral therapy (CBT) is most effective in treating anxiety disorders. CBT involves a relatively short series of weekly meetings with a therapist, with the goal of identifying and changing negative or irrational thought patterns that can lead to dysfunctional behaviors. (The actual number of sessions varies widely and is influenced as much by insurance or health-plan policies as actual patient needs.) For instance, one might not realize how powerfully the need for affirmation and praise drives behaviors that ultimately undermine resilience. During CBT, therapists help patients see these kinds of patterns and suggest ways to interrupt or replace negative or unhelpful thinking with more realistic, positive attitudes and expectations.

CBT can take a number of forms, but all are based on the observation that some dysfunctional reactions or behaviors are learned or, at least, can involve learning. We often associate pleasant or unpleasant experiences with people, objects, or surroundings in which those experiences took place. For people with anxiety disorders, such conditioning can reinforce or amplify the disorder. For example, if you have a panic attack when you cross a bridge, the memory of that experience will powerfully predispose you to having another attack the next time you cross a bridge. CBT often involves relaxation training, a proven and relatively easy-to-learn technique for helping to calm and stabilize the body's fight-or-flight anxiety response in specific situations.

Another form of CBT is a particularly rigorous type of exposure therapy pioneered by David H. Barlow at Boston University. Here patients undergo an intensive series of carefully controlled encounters with the object of their anxiety — speaking in public, for example, or being enclosed in a tight space. This kind of direct confrontation with feared situations may not be for everyone, but for highly motivated patients it appears to work well. Again, no single therapy works for everyone. The key is finding one that works with a person's unique personality and circumstances.

For difficulties with relationships, other types of therapy can be very helpful. Interpersonal therapy is a pragmatic, results-oriented process that typically involves twelve to sixteen one-hour sessions focused on specific goals, usually dealing with relationships. Family therapy can be extremely valuable when children, teens, or other family members have been affected by another family member's anxiety disorder. Family therapy can provide a safe forum for everyone involved to speak and be heard, which can be difficult but also tremendously rewarding.

Bear in mind that the timing of psychotherapy can be important. Sometimes the anxiety disorder must be brought under control with medications before psychotherapy can be truly effective. "When you feel horrible, it's hard to sit down and talk," says Isaac, the man whose panic disorder we described in the previous chapter. Psychotherapy requires energy and attention, which can be in short supply during a lengthy period of anxiety.

Now we'll explore how medications and psychotherapy can be tailored for specific types of anxiety disorders.

OPTIMAL TREATMENT FOR SOCIAL ANXIETY DISORDER

Psychotherapy, various SSRIs, and the antidepressant Effexor (venlafaxine) are usually the first choices for treating social anxiety disorder. The medications can effectively reduce the anxiety, sense of dread, avoidance, and physical symptoms felt in social settings. Cognitive-behavioral therapy is also effective and may suffice for treating specific social anxiety disorder, such as anxiety concerning public speaking. Medications are usually used in combination with psychotherapy for generalized social anxiety disorder.

Some people find they can use fast-acting medications such as the benzodiazepines on an as-needed basis. Also useful are so-called beta-blockers; most often prescribed for heart disease, they can reduce physical symptoms of anxiety, such as a trembling or racing heart.

OPTIMAL TREATMENT FOR POSTTRAUMATIC STRESS DISORDER (PTSD)

Most studies conducted to date on the treatment of PTSD have involved various types of psychotherapy, particularly cognitive-behavioral therapies and group therapy. The goal of these therapies is to help people accept, understand, and integrate traumatic events so that intrusive memories, anxiety attacks, depression, or other physical and mental symptoms can be reduced. Most studies find that psychotherapy helps achieve these goals, though the success rate seems lower among people with PTSD than among those with other types of disorders, reflecting the more powerful influence of underlying biological dysfunctions.[4]

Cognitive-behavioral therapy often consists of both exposure therapy and anxiety management strategies. Exposure therapy aims to extinguish the powerful influence of fear conditioning among PTSD patients. Sustained exposure (usually through remembering and focusing on the traumatic event) can markedly reduce a patient's fear response to trauma-related stimuli as well as the hyperreactivity of the fight-or-flight anxiety circuitry. Exposure therapy must be handled carefully, of course, to avoid exacerbating a patient's problems with intrusive memories. Not every case of PTSD is suited to exposure therapy — the decision must be made on an individual basis by a trained therapist.

Anxiety management training involves learning new ways to reduce anxiety through specific approaches such as the following:

- Relaxation training (conscious strategies to progressively relax muscles and calm thoughts)
- Biofeedback training (using electronic monitors of physiological functions, such as heart rate, to provide feedback to the patient on the effectiveness of his or her relaxation efforts)

- Social skills training (lectures and role modeling of effective social skills)
- Distraction techniques (training that strengthens the ability to consciously distract attention away from unwanted thoughts, memories, or feelings)
- Cognitive restructuring (a gradual training of thinking to correct the tendency of PTSD patients to perceive danger even in neutral and innocuous situations)

At the time of this writing the only drugs specifically approved for PTSD are Zoloft (sertraline) and Paxil (paroxetine). Many patients, however, have incomplete responses to these SSRIs.[5] Other potentially helpful medications that seem to reduce the incidence of nightmares are two drugs commonly used to relieve high blood pressure, Catapres (clonidine) and Minipres (prazosin).[6] Some preliminary evidence supports the use of relatively new antipsychotic medications such as Zyprexa (olanzapine) and Risperdal (risperidone), particularly when used in conjunction with an SSRI.[7] Aside from temporary or short-term use, benzodiazepines are not effective against posttraumatic stress disorder.

One aspect of PTSD therapy that has come under deserved scrutiny in recent years is the effort to recover "lost" memories of trauma, most often memories of sexual abuse or rape; some therapists have encouraged patients to try this. But though some individuals undoubtedly repress or avoid certain painful memories, little research supports the idea that people can completely extinguish powerful, emotionally charged memories only to have them "recaptured," unaltered, years or decades later.[8] The opposite phenomenon is more typical: the stronger the emotion connected with a memory, the more vividly and indelibly it is etched into memory. Much laboratory research has also demonstrated that even very recently formed memories are malleable to a degree not generally appreciated.[9]

Reports of recovered memories, heavily covered by the media a few years ago, may have resulted more from therapy techniques than patients' suppressed experiences. It is perilously easy for clinicians to consciously or unconsciously influence the way patients respond to questions or suggestions. We believe the incidence of recovered memories has been greatly exaggerated, and the resurfacing of completely forgotten trauma is very rare. According to the American Psychological Association, "experienced clinical psychologists state that the phenomenon of a recovered memory is rare." For example, one experienced practitioner reported that a recovered memory arose only once in twenty years of practice.[10]

OPTIMAL TREATMENT FOR GENERALIZED ANXIETY DISORDER (GAD)

The currently favored treatment for generalized anxiety disorder is an SSRI or the antidepressant Effexor combined, during the initial weeks of treatment, with a benzodiazepine, which is then tapered off in six to twelve weeks. As is true for all anxiety disorders, the choice of the specific antidepressant and benzodiazepine is made after considering factors such as age, use of other medications, medical history, and the extent to which insomnia is a significant symptom.

Another medication helpful with generalized anxiety disorder (but not other anxiety disorders) is BuSpar (buspirone). Used for more than twenty years, this medication effectively relieves symptoms of generalized anxiety disorder without incurring the risk of tolerance and dependence. This can be an advantage in patients at risk for alcohol or drug abuse, for whom the benzodiazepines can be problematic. It shares with the SSRIs the drawback of a two-week lag time before a benefit is felt and up to an eight-week period for a complete therapeutic effect to take place.

OPTIMAL TREATMENT FOR PANIC DISORDER

Many studies show that appropriate treatment with psychotherapy, medication, or a combination of the two can reduce or prevent the attacks of immobilizing fear and anxiety common in panic disorder. Most patients show significant progress after a few weeks of therapy. Relapses may occur, but they respond to treatment as robustly as the initial episode. The best-studied form of psychotherapy is cognitive-behavioral therapy, which has been shown to extend and solidify the improvements made by patients in the early phases of therapy.[11] In such cases, psychotherapy and medications are usually begun at roughly the same time, with the psychotherapy lasting from three weeks to six months, after which the medications are used alone. As with other anxiety disorders, the SSRIs and Effexor are now the first-choice medicines, with benzodiazepines used in the initial few weeks while the antidepressant kicks in. The older class of MAOI antidepressants can sometimes be effective when other medications fail, but patients must work closely with their doctor to avoid potentially hazardous food interactions. Some patients with panic disorder find relief with regular use of a benzodiazepine, though the doses required to prevent attacks is usually roughly double the typical dose for other anxiety disorders.

6

THE WORLD OF DEPRESSION

> All his life he suffered spells of depression, sinking into the brooding depths of melancholia, an emotional state which, though little understood, resembles the passing sadness of the normal man as a malignancy resembles a canker sore.
>
> — WILLIAM MANCHESTER, writing about Winston Churchill in
> *The Last Lion: Winston Spencer Churchill, vol. 1: Visions of Glory*

DEPRESSION IS SNEAKY. Unlike panic attacks, which strike swift and hard, depression usually creeps up slowly, sapping vitality, pleasure, and meaning from life while its victims often remain unaware of it until they are firmly in its grip. It's a disease that can strike anyone, regardless of wealth, status, fame, education, or any attributes commonly thought to confer happiness.

Tom Johnson knows this truth all too well. In the summer of 1989 Johnson was publisher of the *Los Angeles Times,* a paper he helped shape into one of the largest and most well respected in the world. But in the decade it took to bring the paper to that height, he stepped on some toes, including those of some members of the family who owned the paper and felt Johnson had pushed it in too liberal a direction. On Friday, June 30, at 3:00 P.M., the family took their revenge.

"My boss called me in and said, 'Tom, I've decided to make a change,'" Johnson says. "It was a clear, clean boot out of a job I just loved. In a single day I went from running an organization of about twelve thousand people to having an office and a secretary."

The boot was disguised as a promotion — to the newly created title of vice-chairman of the board. But the title carried no power — it was simply a platform from which he could look for another job.

Johnson was devastated. Journalism had been his life's work since he had taken a job in the ninth grade at the local paper in Macon, Georgia, where he grew up. He was hired to run in the sports scores from local games, but he quickly learned to type and began writing.

"The moment I walked into that newsroom I absolutely fell in love with it," he says.

Journalism became a very jealous lover.

"I was a workaholic," Johnson says of his decades in the trade. "I had no hobbies outside of work — just a total, total love of what I did. I was out the door as early as I could, and I got home as late as I could. I felt it was a calling, that I could really make a difference in the world. But I missed a big stretch of my children's lives, early on. I was an absentee father, and I look back now with great regret at the time I didn't spend with my children."

Even as Johnson rose quickly through different jobs on his way to the top of the *L.A. Times,* he began to feel a slow and mysterious draining of his energy, verve, and well-being.

"I began to lose interest in everything," he says. "I was enveloped in darkness. I became down, sad, withdrawn. I was *so* tired. I had a little room in my office, and I would just lie down on the floor to recharge. It took a Herculean effort to get myself off the floor and back to work."

He resisted getting help.

"I felt that seeing a psychiatrist or doing therapy was the ultimate sign of weakness," he says. "I had also seen from my time in government service that going to a psychiatrist or getting medication for a mental illness made it impossible to get security clearances. You're labeled, and the stigma is very powerful. I fought getting help much, much longer than I should have."

Finally, at his wife's urging, he sought professional help. In addition to therapy, which he says helped him understand some of the struggles he was having with his son, he was prescribed some antidepressant medications. The drugs made him feel "like a zombie," but he struggled on.

"I was keeping it totally secret from everybody," he says. "I was depressed, angry, and withdrawn. I was so down . . . I was hurting."

When the boot came that June in 1989, he spiraled downward quickly, despite the medication and therapy.

"I thought about ways to kill myself . . . guns, car, jumping," he says. "The medication wasn't working. The therapy sessions weren't working. If my mother had not still been alive and had I not been her only child and sole source of income, and knowing the incredible pain it would have caused her, I would have killed myself."

After a year of constant struggle, Johnson was offered the presidency of Cable News Network (CNN), then owned by Ted Turner. Johnson loved the idea of returning to Georgia and running the all-news channel. But he didn't feel he could do it without being straight with Turner, despite his qualms about doing so.

"I really wanted the job," he says. "But I felt I owed it to Ted to be honest with him. I told him in a restaurant in Santa Monica and the conversation went something like this: 'Ted, before I accept this job, I just want you to know that I've been battling depression.' And he said, 'Hell, pal, let me tell you about me!' And he went through his whole experience with depression."

The day after Johnson started at CNN, Saddam Hussein invaded Kuwait. In the wall-to-wall intensity of the next months of coverage, the depression disappeared. "It was a newsman's walk on the moon," Johnson says. "I was on a high for months."

When he felt the depression creeping back, he sought help in Atlanta and found a psychopharmacologist who tried what was then a new drug, Effexor (venlafaxine).

"My doctor hit exactly the medication I needed," he says. "It took a few weeks, but I really started to feel like my old self. I felt better, and it's really been doing an effective job for me."

After a decade at the helm of CNN, Ted Turner sold the company to Time-Warner, and the pressure began to build for Johnson.

"You're measured by daily ratings and quarterly earnings performance, and you're dealing with very prickly people and some difficult personalities," he says. "And after Ted left, the profit demands started to get unrealistic . . . and I could just feel it all coming back, even with the Effexor."

Johnson was sixty years old, his children were grown, and he was financially secure. He decided to quit before the stress dragged him down again.

"On the day I left I was walking across the pedestrian bridge from the CNN center to the parking lot, and I suddenly felt as though these poisonous spirits were leaving my body . . . I'm serious . . . I just felt them leaving me. I didn't have to worry about budgets anymore or unrealistic targets for earnings, and I didn't have to deal with difficult talent. It was like, whoosh . . . I felt so much better."

Since that day in July 2001, Johnson has split his time between public speaking and writing about depression and reconnecting with his children and his two young grandchildren.

"Do I miss the action?" he says. "Yes. Do I miss some of the people?

Yes. But this is the best stretch of my life, right now, by far. And I attribute a lot of it to getting professional help."

THE FEELING OF DEPRESSION

Tom Johnson's story strikes themes common to many people who grapple with depression: the insidious way it erodes vitality; the day-to-day battle; the futility of wealth, power, or position to ward it off; the value of seeking professional help; and the real possibility for a return to health and greater resilience. Tom also tried to convey something of how depression actually feels. He says he was "enveloped in darkness" and that he was "down," "sad," and "hurting." But these words only hint at the depth of pain involved in depression, a condition notoriously difficult to capture with words.

The writer William Styron calls depression a "true wimp of a word for such a major illness." In his 1990 chronicle of his own battle with depression, *Darkness Visible*, Styron comes as close as anybody to describing the peculiar torment that attends depression, but even he acknowledges the difficulty:

> That the word "indescribable" should present itself is not fortuitous, since it has to be emphasized that if the pain were readily describable most of the countless sufferers from this ancient affliction would have been able to confidently depict for their friends and loved ones (even their physicians) some of the actual dimensions of their torment, and perhaps elicit a comprehension that has been generally lacking; such incomprehension has usually been due not to a failure of sympathy but to the basic inability of healthy people to imagine a form of torment so alien to everyday experience. For myself, the pain is most closely connected to drowning or suffocation, but even these images are off the mark.[1]

If you are depressed, or have been depressed, you know it is awful at best and, at worst, so unbearable that suicide seems perfectly logical. Depression is not just feeling "down," "blue," or "in the dumps." Appreciating the agony of depression, even if only intellectually, helps people be less judgmental, more accepting, and more available to those wrestling with this insidious disease.

Depression renders the sufferer incapable of experiencing pleasure in the broadest sense. Indeed, the loss of pleasure (anhedonia) is its cornerstone symptom. Many other symptoms may also shape a person's particular depression — no part of the mind, body, or personality is left untouched — but anhedonia is at its heart. Some disturbances are easy to see: changes in the way food tastes; unusual sleepiness or, conversely, an inability to sleep; lack of interest in sex; fatigue; and increased pain or sensitivity to pain. But some changes are more subtle, though they may be even more debilitating or dangerous.

Depression makes it harder to perform these mental tasks:

- Think clearly and rapidly
- Concentrate
- Retain new knowledge
- Recall previously stored information
- Reason analytically
- View events from multiple perspectives
- Make decisions[2]

Depressed people often complain of having to reread text in order to get the information to stick in their brains. They are easily distracted, and if they experience a failure in even a small task, they are apt to give up completely or make even more failures as they continue.[3] This cognitive dysfunction exacerbates the depression. With perspective clouded and thinking ability impaired, sufferers can fall prey to an insidious tunnel vision — an illusion that they are thinking and perceiving the world around them with a brutal (and usually dismal) clarity when, in fact, their thinking is warped and out of touch with reality. In its extreme form, this tunnel vision can lead to the conclusion that the only sensible escape is suicide. (For more information about suicide, see Chapter 9.)

It is also true that a person's preexisting cognitive style may affect vulnerability to depression. An important study in 2003 found that people who display a rigid way of approaching the world, a high need for control and approval, and low scores on tests of the ability to think for themselves and believe in the validity of their own thinking all raise the risk for depression.[4]

Appreciating that depression damages cognitive ability can make it easier to understand a depressed person's sometimes baffling thoughts. He or she is most often not willfully stubborn or difficult but simply cannot function at his or her usual level. This can be particularly poignant when depression strikes somebody whose lifework and identity are based on the ability to think, write, or speak clearly. For example, when depression hit Leon E. Rosenberg, M.D., former dean of the Yale School of Medicine, this type of cognitive impairment drove him to attempt suicide:

> I couldn't sleep, I couldn't eat, I couldn't teach, I couldn't even read or write. This had not happened during my earlier depressions and was particularly scary because I had so highly prized my intellectual acuity throughout my life. This progressive, profound loss of cognitive function was the last straw. I became convinced that death would be preferable to being brain-dead, that my family would be better off without me as a vegetable.[5]

TYPES OF DEPRESSION

Three primary types of depression exist. Major depressive disorder (what most people mean by "depression") is the debilitating condition described by Tom Johnson and William Styron. Dysthymia is a chronic and corrosive low-grade depression. Bipolar disorder (formerly called manic depression) is major depression that alternates with periods of abnormally high mood in which a person feels energized, buoyant, and outgoing — sometimes to a pathological degree. We discuss major depression and dysthymia in this chapter, leaving bipolar disorder to Chapter 8 because of its unique characteristics and methods of treatment.

Major depressive disorder is diagnosed when a person is experiencing either a depressed mood or a loss of interest or pleasure and five or more of the following symptoms during the same two-week period:

- Significant weight loss (when not dieting) *or* weight gain (a change of more than 5 percent of body weight in a month) or a marked rise or drop in appetite
- Excessive sleepiness or insomnia
- Agitation and restlessness
- Fatigue or loss of energy
- Feelings of worthlessness or excessive or inappropriate guilt nearly every day (not merely self-reproach or guilt about being sick)

- Diminished ability to think, concentrate, or make decisions
- Recurrent thoughts of death or suicide[6]

If substance abuse or a medical illness causes these symptoms, the depression will be formally classified differently, but the severity and quality of the depression will not be different from the experience of those diagnosed with major depression. We also want to stress that this list is a guide only. If somebody had four of the more serious symptoms instead of five, he or she would still be in serious trouble.

Major depression may strike only once or, more likely, repeatedly at irregular intervals over decades. Occasionally it may consist of a single episode that persists for years. If major depression recurs, it often becomes more serious over time, with less connection to specific triggering events.

Sometimes people with major depression also experience symptoms such as delusions, hallucinations, or pronounced paranoia — a syndrome called major depression with psychotic features (MDpsy). This form of major depression is more common than generally realized — probably 15 percent of all major depression — though attaining estimates of its prevalence is difficult. The diagnosis may be frequently missed because the psychosis may be subtle, intermittent, or concealed.[7] Patients with MDpsy more frequently relapse after a period of recovery, more frequently attempt suicide, are hospitalized more often, and do not respond well to either standard antidepressants or antipsychotics when these agents are used alone. The best results typically come from a combination of an antidepressant and an antipsychotic drug in the context of ongoing psychotherapy and/or electroconvulsive therapy (ECT).[8]

The second basic form of depression is dysthymia, a chronic low-grade condition. People with dysthymia don't usually end up in hospitals and don't suffer the same level of pain and disability experienced by those with major depression. Instead, they are chronically gloomy, usually humorless, and easily irritated.

Dysthymia can, at times, descend into major depressive disorder, though this progression is relatively uncommon. Dysthymia can also be punctuated with periods of relative normalcy or even genuine happiness. Unfortunately, positive moods typically depart rapidly — in a day or two — and never reach heights of exuberance, passion, or ecstasy.

John McManamy, a Connecticut-based journalist who suffered from dysthymia for years before getting a proper diagnosis and treatment, describes it this way:

> If we think of major depression as a spectacular brain crash, milder depression can be compared to a form of mind-wearing water torture. Day in and day out it grinds us down, robbing us of our will to succeed in life, to interact with others, and to enjoy the things that others take for granted. The gloom that is generated in our tortured brains spills outward into the space that surrounds us and warns away all those who might otherwise be our friends and associates and loved ones. All too frequently we find ourselves alone, shunned by the world around us and lacking the strength to make our presence felt.
>
> The symptoms are similar to major depression, with feelings of despair and hopelessness, and low self-esteem, often accompanied by chronic fatigue. This can go on for years, day in, day out.
>
> Still, we are able to function, a sort of death-in-life existence that gets us out into the world and to work and the duties of staying alive, then back to our homes and the blessed relief of flopping into our unmade beds.
>
> All too often, we are told to snap out of it. That the invisible water torture we carry in our heads is our own fault. And shamed into thinking something is wrong with our attitudes, we fail to seek help. Some of us turn to the bottle or illegal drugs. Others seek a more permanent solution.
>
> As I sit here writing this, the term *mild to moderate depression* mocks me. I won't even begin to estimate how many years I've lost to a disorder predicated by the modifier *mild to moderate.*

Because dysthymia is not completely disabling, many people aren't even aware that there is a name for what they feel. They may live their entire lives not knowing that, on average, they feel less energetic, less outgoing, less pleasure-filled, and less emotionally satisfied than most other people. And one aspect of dysthymia makes this disorder particularly tricky: the very traits that can cause pain and suffering can, at certain times and in certain places, be useful. People with dysthymia tend to be logical, orderly, conscientious, and meticulous (at least in some areas of their lives) — all of which can make them valuable workers in certain professions. The disorder can also confer a kind of skeptical realism valuable in particular jobs, such as journalism, political activism, or the sciences.[9]

What's critical in making a diagnosis of dysthymia is whether or not those traits *bother* the person or interfere with his or her life. Some people simply believe that their chronically low mood is their lot in life and never give themselves the opportunity to live a happier, fuller life. Others adopt an "experimental" attitude: they try a treatment, and if it doesn't seem to do anything (or makes things worse), they stop (preferably under their doctor's direction, of course) and pursue other ways to increase happiness and satisfaction with life.

With that as preamble, the official guideline for diagnosing dysthymia is a depressed mood for the majority of days in the past two years; also, no more than two months of that time can pass without the experience of two or more of the following symptoms:

- Poor appetite or overeating
- Excessive sleepiness or insomnia
- Low energy or fatigue
- Low self-esteem
- Poor concentration or difficulty making decisions
- Feelings of hopelessness

While these symptoms describe most people who experience major depressive disorder and dysthymia, a significant subset experience a set of symptoms that don't easily fit into the standard diagnostic scheme. Such people are said to have atypical depression, which is not an independent category but a feature of the existing categories. Atypical symptoms are relatively common — a recent study that tracked nearly six hundred people for fourteen years found that almost 5 percent of the sample experienced at least one atypical episode of depression.[10]

Atypical depressive features include the following:

- Mood variability (subjects are sometimes briefly cheered up by positive events)
- Unusual sleepiness or protracted sleep
- Increased appetite and eating
- Severe fatigue ("leaden limb paralysis")
- Extreme sensitivity to perceived social rejection, criticism, or slight

Atypical features are two to three times more common in women than in men, for unknown reasons. Young people tend more often to experience sleepiness and less often to have severe fatigue, whereas increased appetite and rejection sensitivity are more common in middle-aged patients.[11] Having atypical features of a depressive disorder does not necessarily change how the disorder is treated.[12] Both medications and psychotherapy can be effective, with maximum benefit usually seen when the two therapies are combined.

The Roots of Depressive Illnesses

All types of depression usually arise from a combination of inborn vulnerabilities (genetics or medical conditions such as thyroid gland dysfunction) and the interaction of those vulnerabilities, for better or worse, with life experiences, such as upbringing, education, culture, stress, or trauma. A particular case of depression may arise more from genetics, say, than upbringing, but no depression is *all* genetics, or *all* stress, or *all* upbringing. The multiple roots of the condition mean that using multiple treatment approaches usually works best. As with anxiety disorders, an antidepressant may increase a person's mental and physical energy, making it possible, for example, to cope with the logistics and adjustments of a major loss. Meanwhile, talking with a trained therapist can produce valuable insights into how one may have reacted to the loss or how the loss affected significant personal relationships.

Five fundamental factors are usually at work to one degree or another in a depressive illness: genes, neurotransmitters, stress, upbringing, and medications taken for other ailments. Understanding these basic influences promotes insight into depression and enables more effective collaboration with health-care providers in the search for optimal treatment.

Genes

Depression clearly runs in families. Susceptibility to a depressive disorder is two to four times greater than normal if a person's parents, sibling, or child also has such a disorder.[13] Studies of identical twins (who have identical genes) separated at birth and reared in different families show that the rate of depression in such twins is about 35 percent, compared with the rate among nonidentical siblings of 2 to 4 percent. This strikingly higher rate proves that genes play a significant role in vulnerability. But the fact that the rate is *only* 35 percent proves that genes are clearly not the entire story. If depression was simply a matter of genes, the rate for identical twins would be nearly 100 percent, as it is for physical attributes such as hair color and nose shape.

Researchers are beginning to zero in on exactly which genes may set a vulnerability to depression. For example, in 2003 a team headed by Avshalom Caspi at Kings College, London, found that depressed and nondepressed people exhibited a significant variation in a gene involved with the regulation of serotonin levels in the brain.[14] The study followed a group of 847 New Zealanders for more than twenty years. The rate of major depressive disorder was twice as high among those with the most significant abnormality in the target gene. Interestingly, however, the genetic difference led to a higher risk for depression only if a person had also experienced a number of significant life stressors, such as a job crisis or the unexpected loss of a loved one. The study thus elegantly confirms the message that genes are not destiny — surroundings and circumstances are also important factors in the onset of depression.

Genetic research is turning up some additional surprises. For example, in 2003 George Zubenko and his colleagues at the University of Pittsburgh reported finding a genetic variation that increases the risk of early-onset major depression in women, but not in men.[15] In the future, specific combinations of genes related to depression may be identified and matched with particular subtypes of the illness. If so, diagnostic labels will become far more refined, reflecting actual disease mechanisms. This, in turn, will allow more precise targeting of treatments. Potentially, such labeling could also help prevent depression by identifying those at high risk and giving them appropriate support before symptoms set in.

NEUROTRANSMITTER LEVELS

Decades of research and hundreds of studies prove a link between depression and the levels of three key neurotransmitters: serotonin, norepinephrine, and dopamine. One of the earliest indications of this connection arose during the 1960s, with the widespread use of reserpine, a drug that quickly lowers high blood pressure. Physicians began to notice signs of depression in formerly healthy patients taking the drug, which as a side effect lowers levels of norepinephrine and serotonin. Following reports of increased suicide among patients taking reserpine, doctors began to use the drug more cautiously and to monitor patients carefully for depressive symptoms.

This finding was helpful, but unfortunately, depression is not simply a matter of having abnormally low levels of serotonin or other neurotransmitters. In several studies researchers have artificially lowered the serotonin levels of healthy volunteers who had previously been depressed; most reported feeling depressed again within five hours.[16] Clearly, serotonin levels, for this group, were very important. But when the same procedure was carried out with people who had never been depressed, nothing happened. Even with quite low levels of serotonin, they reported feeling fine, showing that lack of serotonin does not in every case cause depression. This same phenomenon is observed when norepinephrine levels are manipulated: a loss of norepinephrine brings on depressive symptoms for *some* people, and drugs acting specifically on the norepinephrine system do relieve depression for certain people as well.

As noted in Chapter 2, raising levels of serotonin, norepinephrine, or both likely causes a cascade of other changes in the brain, and those changes, in turn, actually alleviate depression for many people. For example, antidepressants raise the levels of certain brain chemicals called neurotrophic factors. These chemicals stimulate the growth of new dendrites and new synapses between neurons. Thus, antidepressants appear to create more "wires" and thus more electrochemical activity in the neural networks underlying mood regulation.[17] The process of building these connections takes time — about the same period that it takes for antidepressants to kick in, which is evidence supporting this theory.

The relationship between a range of neurotransmitters and depression is being aggressively studied in dozens of laboratories, which bodes well for the future. The brain is complicated, and so is depression. As with anxiety disorders, it is very likely that a number of different biological malfunctions can produce similar problems. Consider the analogy of numerous cars slowing down on a freeway. Are they all suffering from the same "speed disorder"? Though they all show the symptom of slowing down, there may be a variety of underlying causes: sticky brakes, a blocked air filter, a flat tire, or running out of gas. One "blanket solution" won't resolve the disorder — each car needs a different approach, though they may appear to have identical problems.

As we learn more about the biological dysfunctions at work in depressive illnesses, we will be able to construct a much more sensitive and detailed diagnostic system and tailor treatments that correct or offset the actual problem at the root of the illness.

STRESS HORMONES

Whether caused by a job, a relationship, world events, financial matters, or something else, stress is an important risk factor for depressive illnesses, including bipolar disorder. Stress triggers a host of hormonal changes in the body and brain, which interfere with normal mood regulation. This stress response is vividly described by the writer Kurt Vonnegut Jr. in his book *Breakfast of Champions.*

> My mind sent a message to my hypothalamus, told it to release the hormone CRF into the short vessels connecting my hypothalamus and my pituitary gland. The CRF inspired my pituitary gland to dump the hormone ACTH into my bloodstream. My pituitary had been making and storing ACTH for just such an occasion, and nearer and nearer the zeppelin came.
>
> And some of the ACTH in my bloodstream reached the outer shell of my adrenal gland, which had been making and storing glucocorticoids for emergencies. My adrenal gland added the glucocorticoids to my bloodstream. They went all over my body, changing glycogen into glucose. Glucose was muscle food. It would help me fight like a wildcat or run like a deer.

As we noted in Chapter 3, the brain and body can cope well with short-term stress, provided that periods of rest or relaxation follow. But the unrelenting stress typical of many twenty-first-century jobs and lifestyles can degrade physical and mental health and may trigger depression in those with an inborn vulnerability.

For example, one of this book's authors, Charles B. Nemeroff, and his colleagues have found that if the corticotropin-releasing hormone (CRH) is injected into the brains of laboratory animals, they quickly show signs and symptoms of depression, including disrupted sleep and decreased appetite, weight, and sexual behavior.[18] Evidence is mounting that CRH levels are markedly elevated in the brains of some depressed patients, which may impair the growth of new dendrites and synapses.[19] Such changes could be the source of the cognitive damage and tunnel vision discussed earlier. Other studies have found that the size of some important brain structures such as the hippocampus (which is vital to memory formation) are smaller in rodents that have been chronically stressed.

Recall that evidence of altered levels of cortisol, CRH, and other hormones have also been found in those suffering anxiety disorders. The discovery that similar changes are associated with depression helps explain why anxiety and depression so frequently coexist.

Upbringing

Adverse or traumatic childhood experiences are strongly linked to depression.[20] Parental neglect, physical or sexual abuse, being the child of a depressed or anxious mother, loss of one or both parents before adolescence, and other negative childhood experiences disrupt the critical process of bonding and attachment to caregivers. That disruption, in turn, can raise one's risk for both depression and anxiety.

Negative or traumatic childhood experiences exert multiple effects. On a purely physical level, uncertainty, fear, or the anxiety of being deprived of attention or physical contact raises stress levels, and the resulting hormonal and neurochemical tides can damage the developing brain and inhibit learning. At the cognitive level, children learn patterns of behavior and responses by observing their parents and siblings. For example, if parents respond to a child's minor injuries with excessive or exaggerated concern and anxiety, the child will come to believe that such injuries warrant heightened fear and, in turn, become hypersensitive to pain or injury. At the other extreme, parents who withhold attention or are simply absent when injury occurs will sow the emotional seeds of abandonment and emotional detachment.[21]

As always, a person's inborn temperament and disposition interact with other people and events. Patterns of emotional response or cognitive viewpoint learned in childhood can carry over into adulthood. For example, a romantic breakup will trigger a much stronger emotional response if you believe you'll never be loved again or that you are incomplete and empty without a life partner. Irrational or overly negative beliefs and attitudes probably do not cause depression in and of themselves, but they can exacerbate the negative ruminations characteristic of depression and block the motivation to seek help.

Of course, childhood experiences can also be positive. Studies with primates and rodents show that physical contact, attention to needs, and exposure to mild, nontraumatic stressors such as peer play "inoculate" animals to subsequent severe stress. In the same way, supportive, caring parents can offset other risk factors that might predispose a person to depression. (See Chapter 12 for more information about anxiety and depression in childhood.) Psychotherapy can be extremely helpful for understanding, integrating, and dealing with troubled upbringing. Doing so may both heal old wounds and reduce one's risk for future depression.

MEDICATIONS

Depression can be an unexpected side effect of many commonly prescribed medications. For example, a young medical researcher was prescribed the common medication prednisone to treat inflammation and tenderness in her hands, resulting from her constant use of a computer mouse. Within days of using the prednisone, the researcher began to lose energy and sink into a gloomy mood quite different from her normal high-spirited personality. Neither she nor her doctor, however, initially suspected that the prednisone was the cause and looked instead at factors in her life — her stressful job, for example, and interpersonal issues with her partner. After two months, which the woman describes as a "nightmare," the pain and swelling in her hands had diminished and she stopped taking the prednisone. Three weeks later she was back to normal and only then, with the benefit of hindsight, did she and her physician realize she had experienced a relatively rare, but significant, side effect of this common medication.

Every day, thousands of people cope with mild to severe mood disturbances caused by medications used to treat some other disease or condition — almost always without knowing that the medication is causing the symptoms.

The list of medications that can induce depression includes some antibiotics, benzodiazepines (such as Valium and Xanax), and drugs to reduce swelling, lower blood pressure, fight cancer, control seizures, prevent pregnancy, and treat acne. (For a complete list, see Appendix III.) Alcohol use can also exacerbate negative moods and raise the risk for a depressive illness.

The young medical researcher's story also shows that even when a medication causes sudden, severe depression in a highly informed person, connecting the cause with the effect can still be difficult. Unfortunately, many of the mood shifts caused by medications are very subtle, making them hard for doctors to detect. Millions of people today have no idea that their medications might affect their mood for the worse, and thus they suffer needlessly.

SEASONAL VARIATIONS IN MOOD

Many animals are sensitive to seasonal changes in light levels. Nature has endowed them with complicated neural machinery whereby the amount of light entering their eyes prompts changes in fur color, the start of hibernation, stimulation of sex hormones that signal mating season, and migration. It appears that humans have some of this same machinery, though its effects are much weaker. Research has shown, for instance, that declining light levels cause an increase in the release of the hormone melatonin from the pineal gland. Melatonin, in turn, influences sleep patterns, body temperature, and appetite. But whether light levels are involved in the genesis of depression remains unclear.

Some people appear to be particularly sensitive to declining light levels in fall and winter. Coined in the 1980s, the term *seasonal affective disorder (SAD)* describes depressive symptoms appearing only in winter among people otherwise free of symptoms. We now know that SAD is both a condition in itself and a potential complicating factor in major depression, dysthymia, and bipolar disorder. Patients with SAD have virtually none of the biological alterations reported by patients with major depression and may, therefore, represent a distinct medical problem. The treatment of choice for SAD is light therapy — regular exposure to full-spectrum high-intensity lights. Light therapy works rapidly — typically within a few days — and can be combined with medications if needed.

TRAUMATIC GRIEF

The writer Andrew Solomon, who has battled depression most of his life, points out in his 2001 book *The Noonday Demon* that "grief is depression in proportion to circumstance; depression is grief out of proportion to circumstance."[22] In other words, grief is a normal emotional response to loss, and although it is characterized by most of the symptoms of depression, such as withdrawal, sleeping and eating disturbances, agitation, sadness, and lack of energy, it slowly passes and does no lasting harm. Grief can actually result in personal growth, greater resilience, and a new or renewed sense of satisfaction with life. Most people go though four stages of grief, though people move through them at different rates:

1. Initial reactions of numbness, shock, disbelief, denial
2. Protest — a period of intense emotions that may include deep sadness or feelings of emptiness, anger, guilt, or fear
3. Disorganization — a period following the acceptance of the reality of the loss, in which a person may feel confused, apathetic, or even suicidal
4. Reorganization — the positive acceptance of the loss, a renewed sense of energy, and integration of the loss both internally and in the logistics of daily life

Most people move through these stages in six months or less, but some get stuck in one of the first three phases and can become depressed. Determining when this has occurred can be difficult because the duration and quality of grief vary so much among individuals. In 1995, researcher Holly Prigerson and her colleagues coined the term *traumatic grief* to distinguish normal grief from a dysfunctional, depressive grief and proposed a helpful guide for distinguishing between the two, shown in the following table.

Criteria for Traumatic Grief

CRITERION A
Person has experienced the death of a significant other and response involves three of the four following symptoms experienced at least daily or to a marked degree:

1. Intrusive thoughts about a deceased person
2. Yearning for the deceased
3. Searching for the deceased
4. Excessive loneliness since the death

CRITERION B
In response to the death, six of the following eleven symptoms experienced at least daily or to a marked degree:

1. Purposelessness, feelings of futility about future
2. Subjective sense of numbness, detachment, or absence of emotional responsiveness

3. Difficulty acknowledging the death (disbelief)
4. Feeling life is empty or meaningless
5. Feeling that part of oneself has died
6. Shattered worldview (lost sense of security, trust, control)
7. Assumes symptoms or harmful behaviors related to the deceased
8. Excessive irritability, bitterness, or anger related to the death
9. Avoidance of reminders of the loss
10. Stunned, shocked, dazed by the loss
11. Life is not fulfilling without the deceased

CRITERION C

Duration of disturbance is at least six months.

CRITERION D

The disturbance causes clinically significant impairment in social, occupational, or other important areas of functioning.

Source: H. G. Prigerson, M. K. Shear, S. C. Jacobs, et al., "Consensus Criteria for Traumatic Grief: A Preliminary Empirical Test," *British Journal of Psychiatry* 174 (1999): 67–73.

People who are experiencing traumatic grief fulfill all four criteria — though, of course, they may still need help and support if, for example, they fulfill only three of the four. Spotting the shift from normal bereavement to traumatic grief is important because people experiencing traumatic grief have a higher risk of suicide, high blood pressure, heart disease, complications of diabetes, osteoporosis, and other physical ills.[23] Fortunately, many effective treatments for traumatic grief exist, both pharmacological and psychotherapeutic. The key is identifying the presence of traumatic grief and seeking help as quickly as possible.

This chapter has explored major depression and dysthymia, two of the most corrosive afflictions of the human spirit. We've seen that both arise from a combination of factors, some biological, some having to do with one's life circumstances. Finding the optimal treatment for these depressive disorders — the subject of the next chapter — usually requires paying attention to both of these fundamental roots.

7

FINDING OPTIMAL RELIEF
FROM BOTH MAJOR AND
LOW-LEVEL DEPRESSION

Canst thou not minister to a mind diseased?
Pluck from the memory a rooted sorrow,
Raze out the written troubles of the brain,
And with some sweet oblivious antidote,
Cleanse the stuffed bosom of that perilous stuff
Which weighs upon the heart?

— WILLIAM SHAKESPEARE, *Macbeth*

RESEARCH SHOWS that more than four of every five people with depressive disorders improve when they receive appropriate treatment.[1] But finding the best treatment — whether medication, psychotherapy, or both — demands patience and commitment on the part of both patient and caregiver.

Two persistent myths continue to limit the effectiveness of treatment: the belief that the first medication a person tries is likely to be the best, and the idea that a single medication is always preferable to several medications. Neither is true.

One of us (Dennis S. Charney), along with his colleagues, found that from four to five of every ten people who try an antidepressant medication will either not respond or will respond poorly to it and thus require a trial with another drug.[2] It can take time to find the medication that works best and causes the fewest side effects. In addition, optimal results are often found with a combination of drugs — a common situation in other branches of medicine, such as the treatment of heart disease. People with heart disease often need several medications because the underlying biology of the illness is complicated, and differences among patients require flexibility in combining drugs. The same is true for depressive illnesses, including bipolar disorder.

Thousands of people today are settling for less-than-optimal treatment because they, and perhaps their clinicians, don't understand these two important points. To illustrate what we're talking about, consider the following story.

Shelia Singleton was a thirty-one-year-old housewife in North Carolina, and things were good.

"I had two children, a dog, a cat; I belonged to the right country club, and I had a husband who was really successful," she says. "I had no reason to be depressed."

That's what she told herself anyway, but her husband knew better.

"He kept saying, 'Something's wrong with you . . . you're crying, you're tearful, you don't want to get up, you've lost interest in doing things . . . I think you need to see somebody.' So I did . . . and my husband was right there by my side," she says.

Her psychiatrist started her on a medication then new to the market, called Merital (nomifesine). "It was phenomenal," Shelia says. For two months Shelia felt like she had her life back again. And then, in light of reports of some rare complications associated with the drug, it was withdrawn from the market.

"That's when all hell broke loose," Shelia says. "From that point on we could not find a medication that would alleviate my symptoms without having such severe side effects that I'd have to quit. So we went from A to Z. Finally my doctor said, 'I don't know what else to do for you.'"

It took years to go from A to Z — years that Shelia moved through in a fog.

"I would get up and take my son to school and then come back home and go to bed," she says. "Then I'd get up when it was time to pick him up and come home and go back to bed. And this went on for six years. It was just awful. It's a long time to suffer. I missed so many important times with my children. I have pictures . . . I know I was there physically . . . but I have so few memories."

Then one day a friend told her about a psychopharmacologist at a nearby university who specialized in depression.

Her new doctor viewed Shelia's depression as a challenge. "He said, 'It may take me a little while, but I'll fix it,'" Shelia says. "He was assertive and aggressive, and started combining medications that had a pharmacology similar to Merital's."

After several months of false starts, Shelia's doctor found a combination that worked: Prozac, a low dose of the amphetamine Dexedrine during the day, and a mild sedative at night. Again Shelia's life regained its color and zest. In 1991 she started speaking at psychiatric conferences about her experiences. That same year she founded the North Carolina chapter of the Depression and Bipolar Support Alliance. She had found a mission and a passion that she had never felt as a schoolteacher, the career she left after she had her second child.

Then, in the summer of 1996, the first of a series of storms struck hard. It began when she opened up the monthly bill for her husband's cell phone.

"I noticed that the bill was several pages thick," she says. "I looked and said, 'My lord,' and realized that all the calls took place at ten at night or six-thirty in the morning, and they were about an hour long. And they all went to this one number."

Discovering that her husband of nineteen years was having an affair was devastating, but things got worse than that.

"I thought he'd say, 'I'm sorry. Forgive me. I won't do it again,'" she says. "Instead he said, 'I like you and I care about you, but I am not in love with you anymore.' So I lost my best friend, my lover, and the father of my children all in one four-hour period. He didn't want to go to counseling. He said, 'I'll go to counseling to help you get through this, but I know what I want.' And I just totally fell apart."

Three weeks later a good friend committed suicide. Shelia stopped eating, lost twenty pounds, and spent most of her time in bed. Her doctor changed her medication, and it helped enough to keep her going through the trauma of moving out of her house with her son and dealing with the legalities and hassles of the divorce.

Four months after settling into her new home, she was seized with intense pain from an obstruction in her intestines, which required surgery, two days in intensive care, and months of recovery. Again, she bounced back. By springtime she was up and around, back at work with the advocacy group, and putting the pieces back together — a process she says was helped by her ongoing psychotherapy.

"Any time you go through depression, it takes away so much from your life that it really helps to have somebody to talk to about it and figure out how you can build it up again," she says. "Relationships are destroyed

... and not just marriages ... you isolate yourself so much that friends move on. Then you start feeling better and it's time to get back in the scope of life, but sometimes you need help to do that."

Unfortunately the storms kept coming. Her mother died of a respiratory infection on Christmas Eve, 2000. Five months later her daughter delivered a baby three weeks early, and Shelia was her major support in the month the baby lived in the hospital. Then a benign tumor in her son's shoulder required several surgeries. In May 2002 a mammogram revealed that Shelia had a tumor in a breast. On the advice of her physician she had a double mastectomy followed by chemotherapy, which left her exhausted, weak, nauseated, and bald.

"I never wore a wig or a scarf," she says. "I couldn't stand those things. I mean, after you've been through some of the things I've been through, being bald is nothing ... It all becomes relative."

Her hair is coming back now, and she's slowly getting back to the office, where she continues to push for greater understanding of depression, better insurance coverage for treatments, and a host of other issues. She says she still "falls apart" at times, and she misses the companionship of her parents and her children. But she keeps going, fueled in part by the conviction that too many others are suffering needlessly from depression.

"Most patients don't respond to the first medication they're given," she says. "Their doctor will ask, 'Are you feeling better?' and they'll say, 'Well, yeah, I'm better.' But they're not much better ... they don't know that on a scale of one to ten, they're not feeling better than a four or a five. I know what it's like to be treated successfully, and once you get a taste of it, you want it back again. I can see now what's possible. I know that if you go in feeling a two and now you're feeling a five, that doesn't mean you can't get to an eight or a nine. Believe me, I know the difference between a five and an eight. And if I can get to an eight after everything that's happened to me, then I think everybody can get to an eight."

PRINCIPLES OF OPTIMAL TREATMENT

Shelia's story offers a number of important principles of successful treatment:

- Medication and psychotherapy are both important for optimal treatment.

- If the first medication doesn't work or produces intolerable side effects, try another.
- Sometimes it takes two or three medications to achieve optimal results.
- Sometimes medications need to be adjusted or changed in response to stressful life events or medical illness.
- Don't settle for feeling just a little better — everyone deserves, and is capable of, a full recovery.

This chapter explores the three basic ways to treat major depression and dysthymia: psychotherapy, medications, and electroconvulsive therapy (ECT). Although we discuss these treatments separately, they are not mutually exclusive or antagonistic to one another. As with anxiety disorders, the roots of depression usually consist of a tangle of biology and life circumstances; hence, the best treatment usually involves medication to address the biology and psychotherapy to address the life circumstances.

A thorough physical checkup is the first order of business when a depressive disorder is suspected. (See Appendix IV for help finding a nearby physician.) Some medical conditions (such as thyroid dysfunction) mimic depression, and some medications produce side effects that do the same thing. Again, although primary-care physicians often prescribe antidepressants these days, we urge you to get a referral to a qualified psychopharmacologist or other mental health professional. (See Appendix V for a guide to the training and focus of the many types of mental health professionals.)

TYPES OF PSYCHOTHERAPY

As we have seen, medications are valuable but cannot give you insight or heal relationships. Such vital steps come only from reflection, thinking, and talking with those around you.

Two types of psychotherapy have been shown in controlled clinical trials to be particularly effective for major depression and dysthymia: interpersonal therapy (IPT) and cognitive-behavioral therapy (CBT).[3] Indeed, a 2003 study found that a particular type of cognitive therapy was just as effective as medication for the general population studied and was actually *more* effective than medications among the subset of patients who experienced early-childhood trauma.[4] In general, the best responses — in this and almost all other studies — came from a combination of psychotherapy and medications.

Both IPT and CBT are brief, results-oriented processes that typically involve twelve to sixteen one-hour interactions with a therapist. Initial sessions gather information and clarify the nature of a person's illness and life situation. With IPT, the psychotherapist then concentrates on the ways personal relationships may have contributed to or been affected by the depression. Communication skills, techniques for dealing with disputes or role transitions, and ways to cope with one's own interpersonal weak spots or deficits are all reviewed and explored as needed. Throughout the process, IPT therapists view their role as a collaborator rather than an authority figure. Several controlled clinical trials have found that IPT can be as effective as an antidepressant in cases of mild to moderate depression.

Cognitive-behavioral therapy focuses on changing negative or irrational cognition (thinking) and its associated behaviors. As we saw in the previous chapter, depressive disorders warp and constrict a person's thinking; hence, CBT directly addresses this aspect of the disorder. CBT helps people identify distorted or distressing thoughts and teaches them ways to counter or change such thoughts. Problem solving and behavior change are constantly emphasized. Symptoms begin to decrease for most patients within three to four weeks of therapy if they have been faithfully attending sessions and completing the suggested assignments between sessions.

With both cognitive and interpersonal therapies, timing is important. Depression must sometimes be brought under control with medications before psychotherapy can be truly effective. As Shelia Singleton says, "I needed to see a little daylight, get a little energy, before I got serious about psychotherapy. You've got to feel like talking before you can bring up any other kinds of issues." Psychotherapy requires energy and attention, and both are in short supply in the midst of depression.

MEDICATIONS

Hundreds of controlled clinical trials demonstrate that the medications used to treat major depression and dysthymia are generally as successful as the treatments used for other medical disorders such as heart disease, high blood pressure, and diabetes.[5] That doesn't mean they are perfect. In nearly all the clinical trials conducted to test various antidepressants, roughly 40 percent of those subjects getting a placebo (dummy pill) have a positive therapeutic response, making it difficult sometimes to demonstrate the effectiveness of medications. Much stronger evidence for the benefits of medication comes from studies that focus on the relapse rate of people who take either a medication or a placebo. A systematic review of thirty-one clinical trials of antidepressants found that, on average, the rate of relapse among patients taking a placebo was 41 percent, compared to only 18 percent of those using a medication.[6] Such research and our own clinical experience convince us that antidepressants do work and are extremely valuable treatment tools, but more progress must be made in the search for better medications.

Of the dozens of medications available, none has been shown to be more effective than the others. Medications such as Lexapro (escitalopram), an antidepressant released in 2002, are no more effective than Tofranil (imipramine), in use now for more than forty years. This doesn't mean the two drugs are equally desirable — they're not. Older drugs tend to produce more side effects or have other undesirable attributes. But in terms of the ability to lift depression, they are virtually equivalent; still, this doesn't mean that all patients respond equally well to all antidepressants. For reasons undoubtedly related to differences in underlying biology, some people respond to one antidepressant and not another. In general, the newer antidepressants are safer and produce fewer side effects than their predecessors do, which is why they are more often prescribed.

Some general principles apply to all antidepressants:

- Patients often stop taking their medications when they feel better, thinking they no longer need them. In fact, feeling better is the result of steady levels of the medication, and stopping usually leads to relapse. For many people, optimal treatment means taking a medication indefinitely.
- Patients who miss a dose should not take twice as much the next time unless specifically approved to do so by their doctor. Double-dosing will not elicit a greater-than-normal antidepressant effect and could be hazardous for those already on a high dose.
- Alcohol and other recreational drugs may reduce the effectiveness of antidepressants or exacerbate side effects. Patients should talk with their doctor before using such drugs.

- Although antidepressants are neither addictive nor habit-forming, stopping or switching medications is best done gradually. *Patients should never stop taking an antidepressant without consulting their doctor about how to safely taper off the medication.*

Given these general caveats, we can now describe each of the most commonly prescribed antidepressants.

SELECTIVE REUPTAKE INHIBITORS (SRIs)

The antidepressants used most frequently in the treatment of depression or dysthymia are the selective reuptake inhibitors (SRIs).

These drugs are selective because they zero in on only one or two of the dozens of neurotransmitters present in the brain. (Some drugs are selective for serotonin, some for norepinephrine, some for both, which is why in this section we use the term *selective reuptake inhibitors* as a broad category; *selective serotonin reuptake inhibitors* is used when serotonin is the main neurotransmitter involved. These drugs work by plugging up (inhibiting) the reuptake pumps that clear out neurotransmitters after they've been released into the synapse. (To review the basic functioning of neurons, see Chapter 1.) As a result, the neurotransmitters remain longer in the synapse and send stronger signals to the "downstream" neuron. The increased neural firing sets off cascades of further changes that alleviate the depression.

All of the selective reuptake inhibitors take time to kick in — some therapeutic effect is usually felt within two weeks, but the full benefit typically emerges after six to eight weeks. SRI side effects, while much less severe than those produced by older antidepressants, can still be bothersome or downright unacceptable. Here are the most common side effects of this class, listed roughly from most to least often experienced:

- Headache (typically temporary)
- Nausea (typically temporary)
- Difficulty or inability to achieve orgasm
- Insomnia
- Jitteriness or agitation
- Dry mouth
- Increased perspiration

More than a decade ago some doctors suggested that some SSRIs, particularly Prozac, might increase the risk of suicidal thinking or suicide attempts for some adults. The concern was based on case reports rather than systematic study, which is weak evidence, particularly because suicidal thinking is part and parcel of the phenomenon of depression. But a special hearing of the Food and Drug Administration and subsequent analyses failed to substantiate these early claims.[7] Indeed, increasing evidence demonstrates the opposite conclusion: antidepressant treatment reduces suicide rates.

Adverse events, of course, can occur after the administration of any drug, antidepressants included, and over the past few decades a handful of patients have experienced some unusual side effects, such as rashes, abdominal pain, agitation, and marked sleepiness. But such reactions are very rare and shouldn't deter people from trying antidepressants; every risk-benefit analysis done to date has shown the remarkable benefits of using these agents. Whenever a troublesome side effect is experienced, patients should talk to their doctor; changing the dose or switching to another medication often eliminates the problem.

The table presents different types of SRIs. Critical information about them is given in the following section.

Selective Reuptake Inhibitors (SRIs)

TRADE NAME	GENERIC NAME
Celexa	citalopram
Cymbalta	duloxetine
Effexor, Effexor XR	venlafaxine
Lexapro	escitalopram
Luvox	fluvoxamine
Paxil, Paxil CR	paroxetine
Prozac	fluoxetine
Zoloft	sertraline

Celexa (citalopram)

Celexa is a selective serotonin reuptake inhibitor (SSRI). The Celexa molecule more selectively targets the serotonin reuptake pumps than most other SSRIs do. It is as effective as other SSRIs and has similar side effects.

Cymbalta (duloxetine)

Cymbalta, the newest entry (2004) to the antidepressant market, boosts levels of both serotonin and norepinephrine. Studies show that Cymbalta appears to have a relatively mild array of side effects.[8] It has been shown to be effective for patients with pain symptoms, which are common in depression.

Effexor, Effexor XR (venlafaxine)

Effexor raises levels of both serotonin and norepinephrine. Some patients, particularly those with severe depression, seem to respond better to Effexor than to medications that work primarily on only one neurotransmitter, though it may also produce a wider range of side effects. Effexor XR is an extended-release version of Effexor which needs to be taken only once a day (as opposed to three times a day with Effexor). Unlike the other new antidepressants, a small percentage of patients develop high blood pressure during treatment with Effexor, predominantly at higher doses.

Lexapro (escitalopram)

Whereas Celexa raises serotonin levels with two chemically similar molecules, Lexapro contains only one of those molecules. This medicine is effective at a lower dose than Celexa is and may have fewer side effects.

Luvox (fluvoxamine)

Luvox is used primarily for treating obsessive-compulsive disorder, but it is also effective for depression. Its actions and side effects are similar to those of other SSRIs. Luvox must sometimes be taken twice a day rather than once a day to avoid side effects.

Paxil (paroxetine)

Paxil is classified as an SSRI even though some evidence suggests that it also increases norepinephrine levels. It is now available in controlled-release form, Paxil CR. Paxil may produce more sedation than the other SSRIs do, which can be an advantage for agitated patients or those with insomnia, but a disadvantage for those who are already feeling lethargic or sleepy. Paxil has the lowest penetration across the placental barrier and least secretion into breast milk of any SSRI, making it preferable for pregnant and breast-feeding women.

Prozac (fluoxetine)

Prozac was the first SSRI introduced and is usually more energizing than the others, which, again, can be either an advantage or a disadvantage, depending on the patient. Prozac has the longest half-life of any SSRI, meaning it is eliminated more slowly from the body than other antidepressants are. Therefore drug levels don't drop much if a person misses a dose, but a longer wait must be factored to allow the drug to clear from the body before switching to another drug. The generic form of Prozac (fluoxetine) is now available and is equally effective, as is a new form that can be taken once a week.

Zoloft (sertraline)

Zoloft is an SSRI that, at higher doses, also increases dopamine levels in the brain, which has an energizing effect; this makes Zoloft a good choice for people who feel "leaden" or lethargic. Like Paxil, it does not easily pass through the placenta, and little of the drug is secreted into breast milk, making it appropriate for pregnant or lactating women.

OTHER RECENTLY INTRODUCED ANTIDEPRESSANTS

Drug companies have introduced a number of antidepressants in recent years that work differently from the reuptake inhibitors just described. These drugs work as well but often produce different side effects and less sexual dysfunction. Each has its own advantages and disadvantages, which are described below.

Other Antidepressants

TRADE NAME	GENERIC NAME
Desyrel	trazodone
Remeron, Remeron SolTabs	mirtazapine
Serzone	nefazodone
Wellbutrin, Wellbutrin SR, Wellbutrin XL	bupropion

Desyrel (trazodone)

Desyrel, introduced in the early 1980s, is frequently added to other antidepressants for patients with persistent insomnia because it is often sedating. It can also lower a person's blood pressure upon standing, which can lead to dizziness or fainting, particularly for older adults. While it produces no sexual dysfunction, a rare side effect is a dangerously prolonged erection (priapism), which often requires medical intervention.

Remeron and Remeron SolTabs (mirtazapine)

Remeron increases neurotransmission of both serotonin and norepinephrine, but not by blocking reuptake. It produces relatively few sexual side effects but is usually mildly sedating, and some patients gain weight during treatment with Remeron. Remeron SolTabs are pills that dissolve on the tongue instead of needing to be swallowed whole.

Serzone (nefazodone)

Serzone acts primarily by blocking one of the serotonin receptors and to some extent blocks the reuptake of norepinephrine. Sexual dysfunction is a rare side effect, and the drug doesn't disrupt deep sleep as some antidepressants can. A disadvantage is the need to take a dose twice daily (most antidepressants are taken only once daily). Serzone can interact badly with certain antihistamines, benzodiazepines, and drugs used to treat AIDS. Patients need to give their doctors a list of their current medications to prevent harmful interactions. In a small number of patients, serzone has been documented to produce severe liver damage.

Wellbutrin, Wellbutrin SR, Wellbutrin XL (bupropion)

Wellbutrin has a unique chemical structure and a poorly understood mechanism of action. It is just as effective as other antidepressants, can be energizing, and can suppress appetite. In a recent study of newer antidepressants, patients who took Wellbutrin reported the fewest sexual side effects.[9] (Bupropion is also sold under the trade name Zyban for treating nicotine addiction.) Wellbutrin SR (sustained release) can be taken twice a day, while Wellbutrin XL (extended release) is taken only once a day.

OLDER ANTIDEPRESSANTS

Two older classes of antidepressants are occasionally used for patients who either do not respond to the antidepressants already mentioned or who, for one reason or another, cannot take one of the newer antidepressants.

The tricyclic antidepressants (TCAs) block the reuptake of norepinephrine and/or serotonin. They also block the action of the neurotransmitter acetylcholine, which produces a set of undesirable side effects such as dry mouth, blurred vision, constipation, memory disturbance, and rapid heartbeat. TCAs act as antihistamines and thus can produce sedation and weight gain. Because the TCAs are potentially lethal in overdose, doctors carefully screen patients for any tendency toward suicide before prescribing these medications. In addition, patients should expect to be regularly monitored by means of blood samples and electrocardiograms to verify that their dose is appropriate and not causing any heart problems.

Although TCAs have been considered more effective than the SRIs in treating severely depressed patients, some newer studies fail to support this view.[10] Common TCAs are listed in the table below.

Tricyclic Antidepressants

TRADE NAME	GENERIC NAME
Anafranil	clomipramine
Asendin	amoxapine
Elavil	amitriptyline
Ludiomil	maprotiline
Norpramin	desipramine
Pamelor, Aventyl	nortriptyline
Sinequan	doxepin
Surmontil	trimipramine
Tofranil	imipramine
Vivactil	protriptyline

Monoamine oxidase inhibitors (MAOIs) block the enzyme monoamine oxidase, which normally breaks down neurotransmitters such as serotonin and norepinephrine after they've been released into the synapse. With the enzyme blocked, more neurotransmitter molecules remain, producing the same type of response caused by the SRIs and tricyclics.

Unfortunately, monoamine oxidase is found elsewhere in the body as well, which can produce uncomfortable or dangerous side effects. People taking MAOIs must avoid eating foods such as aged meats and cheeses, chocolate, and red wine, which contain high levels of the compound tyramine. Eating these foods can produce severe headache, flushing, heart palpitations, nausea, and very high blood pressure. While some evidence suggests that MAOIs may be slightly more effective than other types of antidepressants for treating atypical depression, they must also be taken two or three times a day and can produce undesirable side effects such as sexual dysfunction, insomnia, dizziness, and rapid heartbeat. For these reasons, the use of MAOIs has declined considerably in the past decade.

Although MAOIs are an older class of antidepressant, some new drugs in this group which do not require dietary changes have been introduced outside the United States. In addition, a new MAOI patch, which delivers the drug through the skin and thus has fewer side effects than the agents described earlier, may become available in the United States a year or so after this book's publication.

Monoamine Oxidase Inhibitors

TRADE NAME	GENERIC NAME
Marplan	isocarboxazid
Nardil	phenelzine
Parnate	tranylcypromine

COMBINING MEDICATIONS FOR TREATMENT-RESISTANT DEPRESSION

The virtues of combining medications to achieve optimal treatment have become apparent in the past decade. Although combination strategies have traditionally been reserved for patients with depression that resists treatment, such approaches are becoming more widespread as medical knowledge broadens. Physicians must combine medications carefully, though, with attention to potentially harmful interactions in the liver, urinary system, or brain. But when drugs are carefully prescribed and appropriately taken, patients can experience dramatic improvements. Some of the more common combinations follow.

Antidepressants and Stimulants

Modest doses of stimulants such as amphetamine or Ritalin (methylphenidate) can provide valuable physical and mental stimulation for some patients. Both of these stimulants now come in timed-release formulations, which produce a more even effect. Patients using stimulants should be cautious about drinking caffeinated beverages because the added stimulation can produce unwanted side effects such as tremor, racing heart, diarrhea, or insomnia. Patients prone to anxiety symptoms should avoid stimulants, as should any patient with a history of bipolar disorder.

Antidepressants and Lithium

Lithium is commonly used in the treatment of bipolar disorder, but numerous studies have found that it significantly improves response rates among patients with treatment-resistant depression when added to antidepressants.[11] All classes of antidepressants appear equally effective in this strategy. The positive effects of lithium typically take up to three weeks to kick in, although a few patients respond much more rapidly.

Norpramin and Prozac

The tricyclic antidepressant Norpramin (desipramine) and Prozac appear to reinforce each other's antidepressant actions, and patients in some studies responded to this combination who did not benefit from either drug alone. These conclusions are based on several open studies as well as on a more definitive controlled clinical trial completed in 2003.

Wellbutrin and an SSRI

The combination of Wellbutrin and an SSRI is an increasingly common strategy for handling treatment-resistant depressive disorders. In a 2003 study of this regimen, more than half — 54 percent — of the patients, all of whom showed no response to a single SSRI medication, improved significantly after six weeks on the combination dose.[12] The main side effects reported by subjects were headache and insomnia.

Remeron and an SSRI

Another combination therapy with evidence for efficacy is Remeron (mirtazapine) and an SSRI. Remeron acts on both norepinephrine and serotonin. In a high-quality trial involving sixty-two depressed patients, subjects who got a combination of Remeron and Paxil demonstrated higher rates of response and a slightly earlier response than did those given either of the drugs alone.[13] Interestingly, combining the two antidepressants did not produce greater side effects, perhaps because Remeron blocks two specific serotonin receptors, which may improve sleep and prevent nausea.

Antidepressants and Atypical Antipsychotics

Some recent studies show promising results with the combination of an SSRI and one of the newer antipsychotic drugs — Geodon (ziprasidone), Risperdal (risperidone), or Zyprexa (olanzapine).[14] More research and larger studies are now under way to test these results, but meanwhile, clinicians are moving ahead cautiously because this combination strategy appears effective for some treatment-resistant depression.

LENGTH OF TREATMENT

Many people don't relish the idea of taking a medication for the rest of their lives. Although understandable, we believe this view reflects a misperception of the nature of mood disorders and a lack of appreciation for the value of long-term maintenance drug therapy. Simply put, antidepressants do not cure depression any more than insulin cures diabetes. True, with the help of an antidepressant some people make important changes in their lives that reduce their risk of depression and increase their resilience. In such cases — usually involving mild to moderate depression — slowly tapering off an antidepressant under the direction of a clinician may be possible. But not always.

The general rule of thumb is to maintain treatment for nine months to a year following a first depressive episode, then taper off the dose to see if the medication remains necessary. If a second episode occurs, the medication should be continued for two years before another trial of tapering off is undertaken. If a third episode occurs, the medication should be continued indefinitely.

Even when depression is precipitated by a specific event, such as loss of a loved one, the unleashed biochemical chain of events can lead to long-lasting changes in the brain. These changes can leave a person vulnerable to depression long after the precipitating event has been successfully dealt with or overcome. More fundamentally, depression almost always has a preexisting genetic component, which, even if relatively minor, will not go away.

Studies show that half of those experiencing an episode of depression will eventually have a recurrence.[15] In addition, numerous studies demonstrate that continuing medication treatment greatly reduces the chance of relapse — from a rate of four of every five people among those who stopped medication to only one of five people who continued their medication, according to one large three-year study.[16] We urge you to view depression as a chronic condition, analogous to diabetes or familial high cholesterol, which often requires relatively long periods of pharmacological treatment as well as attention to lifestyle issues to build resilience and decrease vulnerability.

A WORD ABOUT SAINT JOHN'S WORT

Of all the alternative therapies for depressive disorders, the most common by far is Saint John's wort (*Hypericum perforatum*), a yellow-flowered plant used to treat a variety of ailments, including depressed mood. Other alternative or complementary therapies are reviewed in Appendix I, but Saint John's wort has become so popular in Europe and the United States that we feel it is important to review the evidence for its effectiveness here.

The claims on behalf of Saint John's wort (made by enthusiasts both lay and professional) greatly exceed the herb's actual antidepressant properties. A number of nonrandomized, uncontrolled studies show that for cases of mild depression, Saint John's wort is slightly more effective than a placebo (a dummy pill) and produces fewer side effects than some standard antidepressants.[17] The placebo effect, by the way, is actually very powerful in the treatment of depression. In almost all of the studies designed to test the effectiveness of various antidepressants, a significant number of people (up to four of every ten patients) report improvements after using only the placebo. Saint John's wort, in other words, may indeed work for many people, but not because it contains any actual pharmacological antidepressants.

Newer and more rigorous studies have shown that Saint John's wort is not effective for treatment of either moderate or severe depression.[18] The National Institute of Mental Health is now conducting a comparison of Saint John's wort, the antidepressant Celexa, and a placebo for the treatment of minor depression.

If Saint John's wort carried no risks and produced no side effects, we would not object if patients wanted to try it. Unfortunately, Saint John's wort does produce side effects, the most common of which are dry mouth, dizziness, stomach upset, increased skin sensitivity to sunlight, and fatigue. The herb also interferes with the action of a number of other drugs, including some used to control HIV infection (such as indinavir), fight cancer (such as irinotecan), and help prevent the body from rejecting transplanted organs (such as cyclosporine). The most important caution, in our opinion, concerns people with serious depression — if they try Saint John's wort, they will probably prolong their suffering and increase their risk of suicide.

Because Saint John's wort is classified as a dietary supplement by the Food and Drug Administration, it can be sold without the rigorous studies of safety and effectiveness required for prescription drugs. The strength and quality of herbal products are often unpredictable. Products can differ in content not only from brand to brand, but from batch to batch. Information on labels may be misleading or inaccurate. For instance, it is not yet known which of the many compounds in Saint John's wort might be responsible for the purported antidepressant effect. Claims that hypericin and hyperforin are the active ingredients in the plant have been proved false.

In light of all this, and since, as of fall 2003, the NIH research remains under way, we suggest that people avoid Saint John's wort if they want to achieve optimal treatment — even if they feel they have only mild depression. For those who want to avoid traditional antidepressants, psychotherapy has been proved a more effective strategy.

ELECTROCONVULSIVE THERAPY

John Brooks Fuqua has lived the American dream. Born and raised on a poor tobacco farm in Virginia, JB (as most people know him) used his inborn talents and energy to become a business giant, one of the richest men in America, a four-term Georgia legislator, and a respected philanthropist who has given away more than $100 million. JB also battled depression most of his life and only prevailed with the help of electroconvulsive therapy (ECT). Although he kept his depression a secret for many years, he decided to talk openly about it and his ECT treatment in his 2001 autobiography. In *Fuqua: A Memoir,* he says:

> Society has traditionally judged depressed individuals harshly, believing that their problem is due to a weakness of character and laziness. Tragically, this only further limits people from seeking medical attention.
>
> I have been treated with everything that has come along over the

past 50 years, including electroconvulsive therapy. I found ECT treatment to be little short of a miracle. In 1995 I took the electroconvulsive, or shock, treatment and have been generally free of depression since that time. I know that shock treatments saved my life.[19]

Like most people who have modern ECT, JB also uses a maintenance dose of an antidepressant, which greatly improves the chance that the positive changes produced by the treatment won't fade with time. (JB is so grateful for the relief he found in ECT and antidepressants that he and his wife have given more than $4 million to promote a greater awareness of depression.)

Modern ECT is a controlled, painless, brief, and highly effective treatment for both depression and bipolar disorder. Unlike antidepressant and anti-mania medications, the effects of ECT are usually felt within a day or two. Because ECT does not involve a drug, it is particularly appropriate for people who cannot take an antidepressant due to adverse reactions with other medications or because of a desire not to expose a developing fetus.

The ECT procedure is conducted under general anesthesia and with muscle relaxants to minimize overt convulsions. A tightly controlled series of mild electric currents is delivered to the brain via electrodes placed on the scalp. Sometimes electrodes are placed on both sides of the head (bilateral) but often only on the right side (unilateral). Unilateral placements have been shown to produce fewer memory problems or confusion after the treatment, but unilateral application does not provoke as rapid or robust a response in some patients.[20] Some clinicians begin using ECT with unilateral electrode placement and switch to bilateral treatment after about six treatments if no response is seen.

A typical course of ECT entails six to twelve treatments, administered at a rate of three times per week. Although the mechanism by which ECT exerts its effects is unknown, it clearly works. Up to seven of every ten people who undergo ECT for depression get relief — a rate higher than that of any of the available medications.[21] A review of fifty years of research with ECT in bipolar disorder found an average effectiveness rate of two of every three people.[22]

The most common adverse effects of ECT are temporary confusion and memory loss. For an hour after a treatment, patients can be mildly confused or disoriented. More persistent memory problems sometimes occur, and it is impossible to predict which patients will suffer such problems. Well-designed neuropsychological studies have consistently shown that by several months after an ECT series, a person's ability to learn and remember are normal.[23] Decades of research on both animals and humans have found no structural brain changes as a result of ECT. In fact, like antidepressant drugs, ECT increases the rate of new neuron formation in the hippocampus, a key brain region involved in memory formation.

Informed consent is an integral part of the ECT process. Potential benefits and risks and a review of all available alternative interventions are carefully reviewed and discussed between doctors and patients and, if appropriate, family or friends. Where medication has not succeeded or is fraught with unusual risk, or where the potential benefits of ECT are great, such as in cases of depression with psychotic features, the balance of potential benefits to risks tilts in favor of ECT.

On the whole, ECT is underused because of lingering fears often based on misrepresentations of the treatment, such as depictions in the movie *One Flew Over the Cuckoo's Nest*. ECT is also used less often than it might be because of a lack of available treatment centers and clinicians' lack of familiarity with the procedure. But ECT is an extremely valuable treatment option for serious depression and for bipolar disorder that has not responded to medication.

HOSPITALIZATION

Hospitalization is necessary for up to one of every ten people with major depressive disorder because the illness can so overwhelm and disable its victims.[24] When a person presents a danger to self or others, he or she needs the total support and care provided by a psychiatric hospital. Some people check themselves into a hospital, afraid they might commit suicide or simply afraid they are incapable of taking care of themselves. Other people are persuaded by family members to be admitted, and, rarely, people will be involuntarily admitted if they pose a clear and present threat to others or are exhibiting symptoms of psychosis.

The average stay for people who are severely depressed is about a week — enough time to stabilize the situation and begin both pharmacological and psychological treatments. The services offered at a psychiatric hospital emphasize safety measures, crisis intervention, acute medication, reevaluation of ongoing medications, and establishment or reestablishment of the patient's links to other supports and services. Release from a hospital does not mean patients are symptom-free — they usually are not. But they have worked through the acute phase of the illness and can function well enough to continue treatment and therapy while living outside the hospital. In short, hospitalization is an important option and can provide much-needed security, comfort, and support for both patients and those around them.

TOWARD THE FUTURE

The search for antidepressant treatments that work faster, more effectively, and with fewer side effects is ongoing and robust. Hundreds of new medications are tested each year; many work in ways entirely different from the action of the current generation of drugs. For instance, several drug companies are exploring compounds that block the action of corticotropin-releasing hormone (CRH). As noted earlier, higher-than-normal levels of CRH are associated with both depression and anxiety. Some preliminary studies suggest that CRH blockers have an antidepressant effect, though it will be years before scientists gather enough information to prove they are more effective or have fewer side effects than the current drugs.[25] Another intriguing candidate, especially for treating depression with psychotic features, is the cortisol-receptor-blocking drug mifepristone, more widely known as RU-486, the so-called abortion pill. A 2002 open-label study of thirty patients with major depression showed that doses of 600 milligrams and 1,200 milligrams relieved symptoms significantly.[26] Larger clinical trials must now confirm these preliminary results.

A nonpharmacological treatment possibility is vagus nerve stimulation (VNS), a technique developed initially to reduce epileptic seizures. A pacemaker-like device is implanted under the skin in the upper chest, and an electrode is threaded up the neck into one of the vagus nerves, which connect the brain to most of the organs in the body. Mild electrical pulses are delivered by the device twenty-four hours a day.

Preliminary studies of VNS treatment for depression are encouraging. If larger and more rigorous studies confirm the early findings, VNS may become an important option for those with treatment-resistant depression because it does not have any of the cognitive side effects of electroconvulsive therapy or any of the side effects associated with many antidepressants. The major side effects of VNS are slight voice changes, coughing, neck irritation, or shortness of breath, which tend to diminish with time.

Another intriguing development, most recently described in 2003, is that controlled magnetic pulses applied to the head can relieve depression in some people. In transcranial magnetic stimulation (TMS), magnetic fields are focused for several minutes on the right prefrontal cortex of the brain, delivered by a head-mounted apparatus. A study with nondepressed volunteers found that stimulation of the left prefrontal cortex produced short-lived sadness, whereas stimulation of the right prefrontal cortex brightened mood. How TMS works is a mystery, and the small-scale studies to date have produced mixed results.[27] But this area of active exploration illustrates not only that the field of antidepressant research is very wide, but also that we live in an exciting time in the field of psychology — a time that may one day be viewed as a renaissance in understanding and effectively treating these life-sapping disorders.

8

BIPOLAR DISORDER:
DIAGNOSIS AND
OPTIMAL TREATMENT

> Men have called me mad, but the question is not yet settled, whether
> madness is or is not the loftiest intelligence, whether much that is glo-
> rious — whether all that is profound — does not spring from disease
> of thought, from moods of mind exalted at the expense of the general
> intellect.
>
> — EDGAR ALLAN POE

EDGAR ALLAN POE is one of hundreds of creative geniuses now generally believed to have suffered with bipolar disorder (BD), a Jekyll-and-Hyde
disease at once deadly dangerous and surpassingly alluring to many of its
victims.[1] Those with bipolar disorder — formerly called manic-depressive
illness — are often miserably depressed and face the highest risk of suicide
(24 percent) of any mental illness.[2] But they can also experience flights of
creative or productive brilliance that have given the world some of its best
poetry, music, literature, and art.

Although classified as a mood disorder along with major depressive
illness and dysthymia, bipolar disorder has unique biological underpinnings, takes a distinctive clinical form, and responds to different medications than other depressive disorders do. Its distinguishing characteristic is
an irregular cycle of extreme mood swings. The broad diagnosis of bipolar
disorder splits into three general types based on the pattern of the swings.

Bipolar I disorder is the "classic" form of the disorder: the manias are
uncontrolled, often destructive, and more than half the time frankly psychotic. The depressions are vicious, black, and fraught with the peril of suicide. People with bipolar II disorder have full-blown depressions, but their

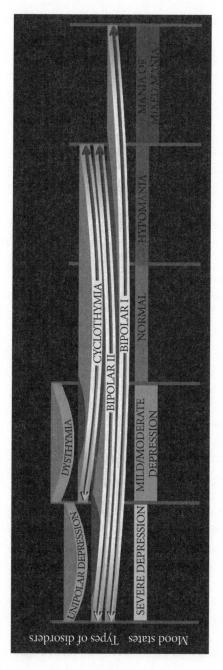

FIGURE 8. *The range of moods.* A person's mood may be normal (center), or it may swing to either increasingly severe depression or increasing giddiness (hypomania) and wild excitation (mania or mixed mania). The moods of people with bipolar I disorder swing drastically in both directions. In bipolar II disorder, mood swings include severe depression, but the "highs" do not reach full mania. People whose moods swing wider than normal yet do not reach severe depression or true mania are said to have cyclothymia. People who typically experience mild but not severe depression have dysthymia, while those who have long-lasting severe depression without swings have major — unipolar — depression. *Time,* Aug. 19, 2002, 42. Copyright 2002, Time Inc. Reprinted with modifcations by permission.

"highs" do not reach the psychotic heights of true mania, being limited to a stage that experts call hypomania, a period of elevated, expansive mood and unusual energy. Cyclothymia (literally, "cycling spirits") is a less severe form of bipolar I disorder: the swings in either direction are less intense, never reaching true mania nor true depression. Figure 8 shows the range of bipolar disorders.

The following personal story, told by Charlene (a pseudonym) and posted in 2003 on the website of the education and advocacy group Depression and Bipolar Support Alliance, illustrates some of the common themes experienced by those with bipolar disorder:

> My father had daily rage sessions and was emotionally abusive. After he finished raging (about anything, it seemed), he would seemingly forget all about whatever he was angry about, and he would be totally jovial and upbeat. He was also alcoholic.
>
> As a child, I thought maybe Dad was demonically possessed. When I studied psychology as a young adult, though, I decided maybe my father had manic-depression. He was never diagnosed.
>
> Myself? Well, I was always moody. As a child, I tended to sit and brood about life. I daydreamed a lot — at home, in class, on the playground. I didn't like reality, so I tried to escape it however I could.
>
> I became a "train wreck" after I left home for college. I suddenly became promiscuous, started drinking and doing drugs, and my first severe depression grabbed hold of me. I remember wanting to just sink into myself and disappear from life. I quit college after the first year because my father died (cancer) just about the time I would have returned to school.
>
> Alas, I continued the drugs and drinking, let a boyfriend move in with me and had unprotected sex that resulted in the conception and birth of a child whom I placed for adoption because I couldn't provide a good home for her at that time. I quit the drinking and drugs after that.
>
> A pattern began. I started jobs, quit jobs, was let go, and my résumé grew. I was chronically unhappy. When I was 22, I had a depression that was the worst I'd ever had. I up and quit my job, moved 500 miles, and continued in a different place with the same pattern.
>
> When I was 24, I went back to college. That was a pretty good time for me, except I overdid things. I ended up working 3 part-time jobs

while carrying a full schedule of classes. I hardly slept, but I never felt tired. I remember one of my bosses at a job told me he thought I should take antidepressants. I got really upset with him. I didn't see where anything was wrong with me. I was doing better than ever (in my mind).

Finally things came to a head. When I was 35, I took a new job at the same time as I was going through a geographical move. My boss at that job was horrible. I began truly losing control of myself. My moods ran the gamut from tearfulness with suicidal wishes, to extreme rage, and to moments I felt invincible and like everything would be all right. But the alternating moods made me feel like I was coming apart. I finally was at my wits' end, and made an appointment with a psychiatrist.

After two decades of being ill and not knowing it, I finally was diagnosed with bipolar disorder. A year and a half has passed now. It took a little while to find the right medications to get me to this point, but I found the right combo a year ago. My friends and family, even my psychiatrist, can't believe the change in me. I found a new job with supportive coworkers and bosses who know about my illness. But I really needn't have told them about it, because I hardly *ever* feel the way I used to. I'm a good employee and I've gotten bonuses and a nice pay raise. And even in those brief moments that I do feel a little maudlin, it's less than half as moody as I used to be. It's nearly impossible to make me angry. What a change!

I guess with money matters, I still have some work to do. Credit cards and bipolar disorder do *not* mix well. But I'm paying off my debts for the first time in my life, and making plans to be debt-free by the end of 2003.

And the timing couldn't be better! My daughter found me online a year ago, and she just turned 18. We're going to meet in person for the first time in November. I'm so glad she'll meet the healthy and sane me.

The manias and the depressions in bipolar disorder often develop over the course of several days or weeks, starting with mood states that are just slight exaggerations of normal.

The hypomanic phase of mania, for instance, is often described by those who experience it as highly pleasurable, productive, and exciting.[3] Ideas come easily and quickly, energy flows, one is possessed with a charisma and enthusiasm that can be both attractive and contagious, and sexuality can be enhanced. The state can be so alluring that even people who have suffered terribly from bipolar disorder can be strongly tempted to quit their medications so they can experience hypomania again. In a very real sense, hypomania is a drug like cocaine or amphetamine except that the active ingredient isn't snorted or swallowed — it's produced in the person's own brain.

In bipolar I disorder, hypomania invariably escalates. Thoughts begin to race so fast that concentration becomes impossible. These thoughts become grandiose, and sometimes paranoid. Ideas are often overvalued ("My book is the best ever written") and sometimes delusional ("The CIA is monitoring my every move because they want to know my secrets"). A severe manic attack can involve vivid or terrifying auditory or visual hallucinations. Judgment is warped even though, to the sufferer, behavior seems perfectly logical and reasonable, leading to spending sprees, sexual promiscuity, and reckless or dangerous behaviors. Mania so reduces the need for sleep that a person may stay awake for days at a time, which worsens the problems with thinking, confusion, and delirium. At its peak, the mania grows so wild and irrational that it is indistinguishable from psychosis, a delusional state in which the sufferer may hallucinate or be otherwise out of touch with reality.

Episodes of mania occur, on average, every two to four years, but people vary tremendously in their cycles.

Bipolar disorder often appears in adolescence — unlike major depressive disorder, which typically begins later in adulthood. Women and men are at roughly the same risk for bipolar disorder, though women have a higher risk for the "rapid cycling" type in which mood alterations occur more than four times a year. Women with bipolar disorder are also at increased risk for an episode during pregnancy and the months following childbirth.[4]

THE BIOLOGY OF BIPOLAR DISORDER

Family studies have long demonstrated a strong genetic component to bipolar disorder. But finding the genes responsible and untangling the related molecular and cellular changes have been laborious. Only recently has real progress been made. As with anxiety and the other depressive disorders, the emerging picture reveals a complicated neural machinery that can become unstable or disordered in many ways. Studies of people with bipolar disorder have found links or associations with dozens of genes, many of them related directly to the regulation or activity of neurotransmitters such as serotonin, norepinephrine, and dopamine.[5] An example of this ongoing work was the discovery in 2003 of a significant variation in the gene that encodes an important nerve-growth factor in the brain (brain-derived neurotrophic factor) in a sample of 136 people with bipolar disorder.[6] Another study in the same year found that a sample of bipolar patients shared a variation of a gene for an important serotonin receptor.[7]

While work continues to clarify the genetic underpinnings of bipolar disorder, other scientists are looking directly at the brains of patients using sophisticated scanners. Anatomical abnormalities have been found among bipolar patients in several brain regions. For example, postmortem studies have found significant reductions in the number of neurons in the prefrontal cortex, which is the seat, among other things, of our ability to control impulses and exert an "executive" role over many other brain functions. Bipolar patients have also been found to have reductions in the number of a certain type of serotonin receptor in their brain stems, which may contribute to mood instability. Size reductions or reductions in the density of neurons have also been found in the hippocampus and amygdala of some people with bipolar disorder.[8] How these abnormalities relate to the genetic findings or to the various patterns of the disease remains a subject of active investigation.

Attention is also being paid to the hormones and brain regions responsible for regulating the body's "master clock." Many body functions follow a twenty-four-hour circadian rhythm — a cycle regulated by pituitary hormones such as cortisol. Studies of patients with either major depressive disorder or bipolar depression have found a variety of abnormalities in the pattern of cortisol rhythms, which probably reflect underlying genetic abnormalities in the control mechanisms of brain structures such as the hypothalamus.[9]

This sample of the many studies and experiments now under way reveals how scientists are attempting to pinpoint the biological basis for bipolar disorder. Much work remains to be done, of course, but as our understanding improves, we should see a continuing improvement in the precision and effectiveness of available treatments.

OPTIMAL TREATMENT FOR BIPOLAR DISORDER

Given the evidence for unusually strong biological underpinnings for bipolar disorder, it's not surprising that psychotherapy alone, though valuable, is usually not enough to bring this disorder under control. The three basic treatments — psychotherapy, medications, and electroconvulsive therapy (ECT) — often overlap and should be viewed as mutually supportive components of an overall treatment plan.

Although not as effective as medications in treating symptoms of bipolar disorder, psychotherapy is nonetheless invaluable. As with other depressive disorders, interpersonal therapy and cognitive-behavioral therapy are the best-studied forms of psychotherapy, and both have been shown to be helpful in bipolar disorder. (See Chapter 7 for more details about these strategies.)

Because BD often involves very disruptive behaviors, therapy often includes family members or other people with close relationships to the patient. Family therapy seeks to reduce expressed emotion (especially criticism) and to enhance the frequency of positive family or marital interactions; in two separate studies it has been shown to reduce the risk for subsequent relapse and rehospitalization of BD patients.[10] Combining family therapy with individual therapy has also been shown to significantly improve and extend recovery. In a 2003 study, thirty people with bipolar disorder were followed for a year; those who participated in integrated family and personal therapy experienced longer stretches of time without relapsing and greater reductions in depressive symptoms compared with those who got traditional treatment. (Patients in both groups were also being treated with various medications.)[11]

A potentially helpful adjunct to both psychotherapy and treatment with medications is participation in a peer-support program. Such programs are increasingly popular because they offer something usually absent from other modes of therapy: direct contact with others who have experienced bipolar disorder themselves. Peer-support groups typically provide structured, scheduled activities such as community work projects or volunteer work for nonprofit organizations under the guidance of a trained mental health professional. Such groups promote friendships, provide information and emotional support, and offer an expanded social safety net that can be invaluable.

As we've noted for both anxiety disorders and other depressive disorders, psychotherapy is most productive if begun after disruptive moods and disordered thinking have been stabilized and a person has enough energy to engage in the therapeutic process. Bipolar disorder almost always requires medication.

Finding the best medication (or medications) for a given patient can take time and effort, but the chances for a full recovery are very good. Often medications are changed based on the stage of the illness. An acute episode of mania, for example, requires fast-acting drugs such as one of the many benzodiazepines or atypical antipsychotics. One of these, Geodon (ziprasidone), is available in injectable form and acts very rapidly, and is thus particularly helpful. Maintaining a patient's stable mood can be accomplished with lithium, Depakote (valproic acid), or one of the newer medications for bipolar disorder (alone or in combination). Before we discuss these medication in detail, consider the following general principles:

- Going off medication can be exceedingly dangerous no matter what patients may think. For better or worse, most patients must sacrifice periods of hypomania to enjoy the stability and sanity of controlled mood swings.
- *Medications must be stopped gradually to give the body time to adjust. Patients should never stop taking a drug for bipolar disorder without consulting their doctors for instructions on how to safely discontinue the medication.*
- Medication may have to be taken indefinitely.
- Alcohol and other recreational drugs may reduce a medication's effectiveness or directly destabilize mood and therefore should be avoided.
- Roughly half of bipolar patients have a concurrent substance abuse problem. Sometimes drugs are used in an attempt to self-medicate the highs and lows of bipolar disorder, and thus when the disorder is stabilized, the drug use may decline. But substance abuse interferes with antimanic medications and makes it harder to control mood, so active treatment and therapy for the substance abuse is usually necessary at the same time that the bipolar disorder or cyclothymia is being treated.
- Regardless of the treatment method chosen, both the patient and the clinician should keep a close record of mood, medications, and other variables such as life events or recreational drug use. Such "life charting" can help clarify how well a medication is working and help pinpoint variables that either improve or disrupt mood.

- Many bipolar patients are extremely sensitive to chemical agents such as alcoholic drinks, topical steroids, caffeine, and some prescription medications. Identifying and eliminating such substances can facilitate treatment.

- Studies show that many patients respond best to a combination of medications rather than a single one.

- Bipolar disorder is often hard on family members and others close to the sufferer. Relationships can be destroyed, finances ruined, jobs lost, and families broken. As noted above, psychotherapy is thus an integral part of treatment. In addition, patient-support groups, which exist in most large cities, can be invaluable for both the people directly affected by bipolar disorder and their loved ones.

- As many as one quarter of all people with bipolar disorder will experience three or four episodes of depression before their first manic episode. Thus they will appear to have major depressive disorder and may be treated with antidepressants. Unfortunately, antidepressants frequently trigger manic episodes in those with bipolar disorder. Both clinicians and patients need to be aware of the following clues that would suggest bipolar disorder in a patient who is depressed, with no prior mania:

  EARLY ONSET. The younger the patient at the first episode of depression, the greater the likelihood of an underlying bipolar disorder.

  FREQUENT DEPRESSIONS. The depressions in bipolar disorder tend to be more frequent and more numerous than in major depressive disorder.

  FAMILY HISTORY. Having close blood relatives with either bipolar disorder or major depression raises the likelihood of having bipolar disorder.

Many medications are available for bipolar disorder, and each has characteristics that may make one more or less helpful for a given patient.

Medications for Bipolar Disorder (Including Cyclothymia)

TRADE NAME	GENERIC NAME
Abilify	aripiprazole
Clozaril	clozapine
Depakote, Depakote ER, Depakene	valproate
Eskalith, Eskalith CR, Lithobid	lithium

Medications for Bipolar Disorder (Including Cyclothymia) *(cont.)*

TRADE NAME	GENERIC NAME
Geodon	ziprasidone
Lamictal	lamotrigine
Risperdal	risperidone
Seroquel	quetiapine
Tegretol	carbamazepine
Zyprexa	olanzapine

Depakote, Depakote ER, Depakene (valproate)

Valproate, an anticonvulsant medication, is also an effective treatment for bipolar disorder. Several controlled studies suggest it works more rapidly than lithium and may be better tolerated.[12] Unlike lithium, valproate is effective in patients with mixed mania or rapid cycling.

Valproate is used both to quell an acute manic attack and for long-term maintenance therapy, though the FDA has not approved this latter use. Potential side effects with valproate include stomach upset, nausea, weight gain, tremor, sedation, and hair loss. Controversy exists over whether valproate increases the frequency of multiple ovarian cysts (polycystic ovary syndrome) in women of reproductive age, a condition associated with a significant reduction in fertility.[13]

People with bipolar disorder are at higher-than-normal risk for migraine headaches, obsessive-compulsive disorder (OCD), panic disorder, and attention deficit/hyperactivity disorder. Valproate is specifically beneficial for migraine and possibly for panic attacks and OCD, and so is preferred in such cases.

Eskalith, Eskalith CR, Lithobid (lithium)

As was the case with many drugs used to treat mental illnesses today, lithium's ability to tame bipolar disorder was discovered by accident. In 1948 the Australian physician John Cade was experimenting with guinea pigs and noticed that injections of lithium made the animals lethargic. On a hunch, he tried lithium on his manic patients. Within a week their mania began to abate, to the delight of both the patients and Cade.

Cade published his results in an Australian medical journal, where they were largely ignored until two Danish psychiatrists read about them in 1954 and replicated Cade's findings. As successful as lithium was, it took a long time to catch on, in part because, as a simple salt compound, it could not be patented and thus was not viewed as a profitable drug. It wasn't until the 1970s that lithium was marketed in the United States. Lithium is now the "gold standard" therapy for treating bipolar disorder.[14] It is more effective at calming mania than in reversing depression, but its overall effectiveness is impressive. Lithium is less effective for certain subsets of bipolar patients, however, such as those with mixed mania (mania existing at the same time as depression) and rapid-cycling patients (those whose manic-depressive cycles happen more than four times a year).[15]

Patients on lithium need to have their lithium levels and thyroid function monitored regularly to ensure optimal dosing and avoid adverse effects. The anti-manic effects of lithium typically kick in after two to three weeks. Possible side effects include stomach upset, tremor, metallic taste, and a perceived dulling of thinking ability. Careful adjustment of dosage can often reduce these side effects. Kidney function must be monitored every six months because lithium can occasionally cause kidney failure.

Lamictal (lamotrigine)

The anticonvulsant Lamictal is approved by the FDA for the prevention of recurring episodes of both mania and depression in bipolar patients. It is particularly effective for treating the depressive phase of bipolar disorder but is less effective against acute mania.[16] As with antidepressants, Lamictal may worsen symptoms of mania in some individuals and, thus, must be used cautiously. Lamictal must be started at a low dose and slowly increased, which is one reason it may be ineffective for treating acute mania.

Possible side effects include headache, nausea, double vision, dizziness, and muscle incoordination. A skin rash occurs in up to one of every twenty patients early in treatment. Rashes are more common in the elderly. In most cases, the rash is mild and subsides spontaneously, but in some patients it becomes a serious dermatological condition requiring immediate medical attention.

Tegretol (carbamazepine)

Tegretol is another anticonvulsant used for treating bipolar disorder, though it is not approved by the FDA for this use. It is generally effective in calming mania but appears to be less effective than lithium for long-term maintenance therapy.[17] Some studies show that the combination of Tegretol and lithium is more effective than either medication used alone.

Tegretol is broken down in a complicated way by the body, which requires close monitoring with blood samples to ensure a therapeutic dose. In addition, Tegretol can increase the breakdown of several other types of drugs such as oral contraceptives, some antidepressants, anticonvulsants, and benzodiazepines. Possible side effects include stomach upset, sedation, double vision, low blood-sodium levels, and dulled thinking ability.

Antipsychotic Medications for Mania

Newer, so-called second-generation antipsychotic medications have been shown to effectively dampen acute mania and enhance the effectiveness of lithium or valproate in some patients.[18] Abilify (aripiprazole), Geodon (ziprasidone), Risperdal (risperidone), Seroquel (quetiapine), and Zyprexa (olanzapine) have all been shown effective in the treatment of acute mania and are useful in maintenance treatment as well. Clozaril (clozapine) may be helpful for patients with a particularly resistant form of the disorder.

COMBINING MEDICATIONS

Many people with bipolar disorder are treated with a combination of medications, either on a short- or long-term basis. Several studies show that combining lithium or valproate with one of the antipsychotic medications mentioned above improves effectiveness. Combining medications sometimes produces more side effects than using either drug alone, but these can be limited by adding the second drug slowly and gradually raising the dose.

ANTIDEPRESSANTS FOR THE TREATMENT OF BIPOLAR DEPRESSION

Another class of medicines that can help people with bipolar disorder is the antidepressants, though these must be used cautiously because they can trigger mania. Nonetheless, for some patients, antidepressants, primarily the SSRIs, provide valuable relief of depressive symptoms after symptoms of mania have been controlled, as long as the antidepressant is used in combination with a mood-stabilizing medication.[19] Side effects are generally less severe than with older classes of antidepressants, but they can still be bothersome or downright unacceptable. Side effects should always be discussed with a doctor since changing the dose or switching to another medication can sometimes help.

The SSRIs that may be effective for bipolar patients are the same as those discussed more fully in Chapter 7. One antidepressant, Wellbutrin (bupropion), is effective in the treatment of bipolar depression and has little propensity to "switch" a patient into mania.

OTHER TREATMENT OPTIONS

As detailed in Chapter 7, modern electroconvulsive therapy (ECT) is safe, painless, and as effective for bipolar disorder as it is for major depression. A review of fifty years of research with ECT in bipolar disorder found an average effectiveness rate of 66 percent.[20] Unlike medications, the therapeutic effects of ECT are usually evident within a day or two. Because ECT does not involve a drug, it is particularly appropriate for people who cannot take medications due to adverse reactions or a desire not to expose a developing fetus. ECT can be used for treatment-resistant mania or depression, and a recent review of the relevant literature in 2003 found "overwhelming" evidence for the effectiveness of ECT in this population.[21] So-called maintenance sessions of ECT, extending a year or longer after the initial sessions, have been found to reduce relapse and rehospitalization rates.[22]

Regardless of the treatment option chosen, a brief stay at a psychiatric hospital can greatly facilitate recovery. About 85 percent of people with bipolar disorder are hospitalized at some point in their lives because of the overwhelming nature of the illness.[23] Mania, in particular, can render a person highly agitated, violent, or hallucinating. Because of potential harm to self or others, a stay in a psychiatric hospital may be well advised to stabilize and support the patient.

The average length of stay for people admitted for acute mania is about two weeks. As with hospitalization for people with severe depression, when patients leave the hospital they are not usually symptom-free. But they will be out of immediate danger and can continue treatment and therapy while living in the community. In short, hospitalization can give much-needed security, comfort, and support for both patients and those around them.

Research to find ever more effective treatments for bipolar disorder continues at an accelerating pace. Combined with the gradual lessening of the stigma surrounding mental illness in general and a rise in awareness of and education about bipolar disorder in particular, those suffering with this disorder have good reason to be optimistic.

9

REDUCING THE
RISK OF SUICIDE

Suicide is a permanent solution to a temporary problem.

— ART BUCHWALD, columnist and depression survivor

ELIZABETH CLAY TERRY first tried to kill herself when she was twenty years old. She was Phi Beta Kappa at Florida State University, majoring in English and government, with a 3.75 grade point average. Her good looks, intelligence, and down-to-earth sense of humor made her a popular and attractive junior. But beneath the apparent confidence and success was a gaping hole in her self-esteem that left her vulnerable to easy infatuation with men.

"Over and over I would fall for some man and believe he was the one who was going to save me, change me, change things around me, and that I was going to be okay," she says. "I had sampled drugs, tried liquor . . . they didn't do anything for me. But men . . . they were going to save me. So I fell in love with this married professor, and although he ended up leaving his wife eventually, he didn't do it for me. And when I realized we weren't driving off into the sunset, I tried to kill myself."

She swallowed a small pile of sleeping pills on a day her roommate planned to be gone. But car trouble brought her roommate back early. She found Clay (she uses her middle name) and took her to the emergency room, where Clay vomited repeatedly and had her stomach pumped.

Despite the obviousness of the suicide attempt, nobody at the university or hospital took further action after she recovered.

"They just gave me the typical talk," she says. "They said, 'Oh, you're such a smart, beautiful young lady with your whole life ahead of you — why would you want to kill yourself?' They just couldn't understand."

Clay knew what the doctors failed to recognize: she was depressed and had been fighting depression despite a happy childhood in a relatively stable family. Looking back, she believes she inherited a predisposition to depression from her mother's side of the family. But at the time all that mattered was trying to escape from the crushing sense of futility that accompanied her depressive bouts.

"When you're depressed, you just feel there is no hope, period," she says. "If you're rich, you see yourself as poor. If you're beautiful, you see yourself as ugly. If you're smart, you think you're stupid. You could be the most glorious human being or you could be a damned homeless person shuffling down the street, and you don't see a difference. It doesn't matter. So you might as well just kill yourself because why in the hell do you want to drag through life like that day after day?"

Clay battled depression for the next twenty years. She was never diagnosed and never treated. She continued to feel suicidal at times and at one point tried to kill herself with an overdose of heroin. Life, meanwhile, dealt her some bad cards.

On the night of April 25, 1992, she was mugged by two men as she was leaving her apartment. She fought and screamed, and the attackers left her when a neighbor came running, but not before leaving her with head and face injuries so severe the doctors were surprised she was not dead, thought she would lose an eye, and felt certain she would be brain-damaged.

Five operations over the next year saved her eye and reconstructed her face and head so perfectly that only a faint scar on her temple betrays the attack.

In the depression following the attack, Clay finally sought help. On the advice of friends she sought out a psychopharmacologist at a nearby hospital. On her first meeting she cut right to the chase.

"I said, 'Look, you need to understand a few things,'" she says. "'First, I am not going to hang around very long. If I don't see some results in a month, well, after that, pal, I'm outta here, and I mean to the next life. I've dragged it around for over twenty years and I'll be damned if I drag it around much more. Second, I want to be able to contact you any time, day or night. If things are bad, I want to talk to you. I don't want to get an answering service.' He said, 'Okay, but now you have to have an agreement with me: if you feel like you're going to kill yourself, you don't do a thing until you have talked to me.' That was our agreement and I've always honored it."

In that first session, Clay scored twenty-nine on a depression-symptom severity scale, indicating severe depression. Her psychiatrist put her on an SSRI antidepressant, then switched after two weeks to Effexor (venlafaxine). Several weeks later Clay's depression began to lift.

"I felt like a new person," she says. "It was absolutely amazing. He retested me and I was at seventeen, and the next time he tested me I was at five. It was wonderful."

Her suicidal thoughts disappeared for a while, and she felt better than she could remember feeling since childhood. But then a series of losses hit like so many waves. Hurricane Opal severely damaged the resort her parents had built and run for nearly fifty years. She lost the job she'd had for a decade with AT&T when the company downsized and laid off 17,000 employees worldwide. Her sister's new husband, only thirty, died of metastatic melanoma. And her beloved Akita dog died. Despite the Effexor, she became determined to kill herself. She had a .38-caliber revolver and was ready to shoot herself around noon one day in the kitchen of her sister's house.

"I just couldn't take any more," she says. "I didn't want any more pain. I was tired of pain. But I called my doctor first because I told him I would. He was God knows where, some foreign country, and it was the middle of the night, but it didn't matter. He was right there. He said, 'Clay, don't you do it or I'll haunt you, and you know, my mother's up there and I'll get her after you, and what is your sister going to do when she finds out?' And I said, 'Oh my God, she'll just yank me right back to this life and beat me into the next one.'"

The conversation was longer than that, of course, but being able to talk to someone who had developed a relationship with her and who could penetrate her faulty reasoning made all the difference.

"Day to day, the pills are wonderful," she says. "I need them. But what saves you is a person, not a pill. When you're desperate and your world is gone and you're sitting there wondering whether to shoot yourself or take the sleeping pills, you don't reach out and call your medication. Effexor doesn't save you. Your therapist saves you."

Since that time, Clay says she hasn't come close to suicide again. She has problems . . . she still can't find a stable job in her field, for instance. But she's able to deal with these issues without descending into depression or suicidal thoughts.

"For the past two or three years I've been cured of the desire to kill myself," she says. "I know that if things get bad, I'll come out on the other end and be okay. That's a pretty amazing thing, for someone who spent most of a lifetime trying to figure out how to exit the planet."

WHY DO PEOPLE KILL THEMSELVES?

Suicide is a symptom, not a disease. But the mental and physical dysfunctions at the root of suicide or a suicide attempt are often hidden. Like the clinicians who wondered why twenty-year-old Clay Terry swallowed a handful of sleeping pills, those closest to a suicide victim are often the most perplexed by the seemingly senseless act.

In truth most suicides *are* senseless. Suicide usually is the tragic final step in a long-standing cascade of mental illness that robs its victims of perspective and meaning. Things look quite different, of course, to most people seriously contemplating suicide. In the grip of depression or some other intense emotional pain, logic and reason become so warped that death seems both unavoidable and desirable. Writer Alfred Alvarez points this out in his classic book on suicide, *The Savage God:* "The logic of suicide is different. Once a man decides to take his own life he enters a shut-off, impregnable but wholly convincing world where every detail fits and each incident reinforces his decision. The logic of suicide creates a tunnel vision, what psychologists call 'constriction.' In this rigid thinking, all roads lead to only one choice, there are no alternatives, no other answers."[1]

Generalizations about the reasons people try to kill themselves are hazardous because people and their motives are complicated. But, broadly speaking, suicide usually arises from one, or a combination, of the following:

- Hopelessness, desperation, or intense emotional pain engendered by major depressive disorder or bipolar disorder
- Pent-up hostility, loneliness, humiliation, or shame
- Distorted beliefs about one's self and one's circumstances caused by substance abuse, schizophrenia, or a mood disorder
- Unbearable physical pain associated with a debilitating illness
- Loss of meaning in life

We will not focus on suicide arising from unbearable pain. We agree with surgeon and acclaimed writer Dr. Sherwin Nuland who wrote in *How*

We Die, "Taking one's own life is almost always the wrong thing to do. There are two circumstances, however, in which that may not be so. Those two are the unendurable infirmities of a crippling old age and the final devastations of a terminal disease."[2]

Unfortunately, most suicides are not rational responses to horrendous end-of-life situations; they are irrational responses to life situations horrendous only because an underlying mental illness distorts and constricts one's perspective and interferes with normal abilities to surmount problems. For example, consider the following suicide notes or excerpts from notes:

> *Dear Betty:*
>   *I hate you.*
>   *Love,*
>   *George*

> *. . . I tried to do my stuff, but after Marshall's summing up, I've given up all hope. The car needs oil in the gear-box, by the way.*

> *There's only one genius in a number of generations. My father is it. The next one can't be expected for 100 years. I've tried to live up to it. I can't. He ranks. I don't.*

> *My dearest,*
> *I have taken my life in order to provide capital for you. The IRS and its liens which have been taken against our property illegally by a runaway agency of our government have dried up all sources of credit for us. So I have made the only decision I can.*[3]

The limited, sometimes quirky logic of such notes arises from the cognitive distortions wrought by a depressive illness. Research suggests that roughly one out of every twenty people — about 4 percent — of the U.S. population will attempt suicide at some point in their lives.[4] Among those with major depression, however, the rate is more than one out of every four people — 27 percent. Numerous studies have shown clear associations between adverse childhood events and increased likelihood of suicide attempts from the teen years on. One recent study found that the following factors were particularly significant:

- Emotional abuse
- Physical abuse
- Sexual abuse
- Psychologically ill household member
- Incarcerated family member
- Battered mother
- Substance abuse in home
- Parents separated or divorced[5]

Assessing the actual number of people who attempt suicide every year is surpassingly difficult because the act can be concealed relatively easily, even when it results in a visit to an emergency room. Research indicates that eight to twenty-five people try to kill themselves for every one who succeeds. This means that in the year 2000 (the latest year for which figures were available at the time of this writing), when 29,350 people killed themselves, between 234,800 and 733,750 people attempted suicide.[6] Most of these "attempters" are women: three women try to kill themselves for every man who does so. Men, however, are much more "successful" in their attempts: about three of every four suicides in any given year are men.

To put the suicide rate in perspective, three people kill themselves (on average) in the United States every hour of every day — almost twice as many deaths as occur from homicide and more than twice as many deaths as occur from AIDS. Keep in mind, too, that available statistics undoubtedly underestimate the true extent of suicide by an unknown amount. Some single-car "accidents," "inadvertent" drug overdoses, and "gun-cleaning mishaps," for instance, are certainly suicides.

Psychiatrists often distinguish between impulsive suicides, in which the sufferer is usually young and responds to a wave of sudden despair, and nonimpulsive suicides, which result from more methodical, planned behavior. Impulsive suicides are defined as those occurring within five minutes of the decision to take one's life.[7] Roughly a quarter of suicides are estimated to be impulsive, with the risk higher among males and those recently in a fight or with behavior disorders linked to impulse control. An inability to control impulses likely is rooted in biology. For example, people with poor impulse control tend to have lower-than-normal levels of serotonin in their brains.[8] Interestingly, current studies have not found any significant differences in the use of alcohol or other drugs between impulsive and nonimpulsive suicide attempters.

As the chart below illustrates, the overall suicide rate increases steadily with age — older people kill themselves far more often than younger people do. But this statistic masks the grim reality of youth suicide. The rate of suicide among the young has been rising in recent decades. Suicide is the third leading cause of death among teenagers (behind accidents and homicide) and the second leading cause of death among those twenty-five to thirty-four years old (behind accidents). Almost four thousand young people killed themselves in the year 2000 in the United States.

With the arguable exception of end-of-life suicide by rational individ-

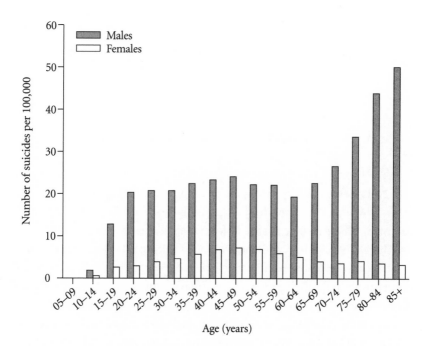

FIGURE 9. *Rates of suicide among men and women in the United States in 2000.* Note that in all age groups the suicide rate for men is much higher than it is for women, and the rate for men rises steeply late in life, whereas the rate for women declines slightly. Data from the Centers for Disease Control and Prevention, National Center for Health Statistics.

uals in severe physical distress, none of these thousands of people should have died. Such deaths are preventable and represent failure at virtually all levels of society to address the foundations of psychological illnesses. Suicide is not an inevitable feature of the human condition, a fact demonstrated by the wide variations in international suicide rates. Consider the information in the table below.

COUNTRY	SUICIDE RATE PER 100,000 PEOPLE (YEAR DATA WERE GATHERED)
Lithuania	46 (2000)
Estonia	34 (1999)
Hungary	33 (2000)
Japan	25 (1999)
Finland	23 (1999)
Belgium	22 (1995)
Canada	12.3 (1997)
United States	11 (2000)
Brazil	4.2 (1995)
Mexico	3.2 (1995)
Philippines	2.1 (1993)
Kuwait	1.6 (2000)
Iran	0.2 (1991)

Source: World Health Organization, *Figures and Facts About Suicide* (Geneva: WHO, 2003).

Nobody knows why such great disparities exist. Religion undoubtedly plays a role, as evidenced by the generally low suicide rates in Muslim countries, where suicide is strictly forbidden and is viewed as a profound sin. But the Philippines and Mexico are not primarily Muslim countries, and they, too, have low suicide rates. Long, dark winters may contribute to the generally high suicide rates in Scandinavia, but Japan, which has a temperate climate, has a higher suicide rate than does Finland. Ready access to guns, which are the most lethal of suicide methods, undoubtedly affects the "success rate" of suicide attempters, but the United States, which has minimal gun-control laws and more than 76 million privately owned handguns, has a lower suicide rate than Canada, which has tough gun-control laws and only about one million privately owned guns.[9]

Clearly, cultural norms, religion, societal expectations, and other factors affect suicidal behavior. But biology is at work as well. The suicide rate among members of the biological families of suicide victims is significantly higher than that of families without a suicide victim.[10] The relationship between genes and suicide was explored rigorously in a study comparing the suicide rate in identical twins with that of fraternal twins, who are no more genetically similar than any two siblings. Of 188 pairs of identical twins, twenty-two of the pairs had both committed suicide (not at the same time). Not a single pair of 254 fraternal twins did so. Genes are clearly involved, but they clearly do not tell the whole story. Note that in that same study, in the vast majority of cases (81 percent), when one identical twin committed suicide, the other did *not*, despite their identical genes.

Researchers have begun to find clues about how genes might contribute to suicide risk. As we have already noted, the brains of suicide victims, especially those who act impulsively, tend to have lower levels of serotonin (as measured by a serotonin breakdown product in spinal fluid) than the brains of people who have not killed themselves.[11] Low serotonin levels have been linked to both depression and impulsive, aggressive behavior, which may contribute to the ability to kill oneself. In addition, alterations in the neurotransmitters norepinephrine, dopamine, and CRH have been found in the brains of both suicide victims and those who attempted suicide.

For example, when normal individuals are given a drug that stimulates dopamine receptors, their brains release growth hormone. But this response is markedly blunted in depressed patients who have previously attempted suicide and in those who go on to commit suicide, suggesting some kind of dysfunction in the brain circuitry supported by dopamine. In addition, the hypothalamic-pituitary-adrenal (HPA) axis (see Chapter 4) in suicide victims is often hyperactive, which may reflect depression, exposure to early trauma, high current stress levels, or some other dysregulation.[12]

Exactly how these brain changes affect vulnerability to suicide is still being investigated, but some research with antidepressants is confirming that the links are real, particularly between serotonin and suicide. A recent study from Australia found that suicide rates declined in areas of the country with the highest rates of prescriptions for the SSRI class of antidepressants.[13] The authors of this study caution that the suicide reduction was probably related to both the antidepressant use and the increased attention given to patients by the prescribing doctors. But other research strongly suggests that raising serotonin levels reduces suicide risk.[14]

Lithium markedly reduces suicide risk in patients with bipolar disorder — and it is more effective than Depacon, Depakene, Depakote, and other trade-name drugs containing valproate as their active ingredient.[15] For patients with schizophrenia, the antipsychotic drug Clozaril (clozapine) has been shown to reduce suicide attempts.

The bottom line: suicide risk can be lowered with certain drugs, proving that suicide has biological underpinnings that interact with psychological, social, and cultural forces.

WARNING SIGNS

It's both possible and critical to spot warning signs of suicide. Here are the most important:

- VERBAL SUGGESTIONS OF SUICIDE INTENT OR HINTS OF SUCH AN ATTEMPT. Statements such as "You'd be better off without me" or "I can't take much more of this" should be taken seriously, particularly if other risk factors exist, such as a history of depression or substance abuse. Contrary to myth, most people who commit suicide talk about their plans either explicitly or implicitly. Also untrue is the notion that if people talk about committing suicide, they won't actually do it. People rarely talk about suicide if they haven't been thinking about it seriously — and that is cause for concern.

- ABSOLUTIST LANGUAGE. The constricted thinking typical of suicide victims leads them to use words such as *always, never, only,* and *forever.* Statements such as "Only Mom loved me" reflect an inability to see alternative possibilities or take a wide perspective on life.

- A PREVIOUS SUICIDE ATTEMPT. Roughly half of those who succeed in killing themselves made previous attempts.[16]

- MAJOR CHANGE IN BEHAVIOR OR PERSONALITY. People who have been depressed may suddenly seem happier, often because they are relieved to have made up their mind to kill themselves. Alternatively, normally cheerful people may become quiet and withdrawn and stop formerly pleasurable activities.

- ALTERED SLEEP PATTERNS. These may involve either insomnia or excess sleep.

- GIVING AWAY VALUED POSSESSIONS.

- RECKLESS BEHAVIOR. Driving too fast, having unprotected sex, or abusing drugs can be signs of apathy about life.
- DEPRESSION OR RECENT EMERGENCE FROM DEPRESSION. Sometimes severely depressed people lack the energy to kill themselves and, thus, paradoxically, can be at highest risk as they begin to recover and gain energy.

IN AN EMERGENCY

Facing somebody intent on killing himself or herself can be terrifying and confusing, but in such cases you may be all that stands between a life wasted and a life reclaimed. The following guidelines may help maximize the chances that a person can be pulled back from the brink of suicide.

- TAKE THE ATTEMPT SERIOUSLY. Do not deny or minimize an attempt, even if you think it isn't serious. This situation is always serious, and consistently maintaining that belief sends an important message to the person threatening suicide.
- CONFIRM. If unsure whether observed behavior suggests suicide, the best approach is to ask directly, using questions such as these: "Have you ever thought about killing yourself?" "Do you have a plan?" "Are you thinking about killing yourself now?" Asking such questions will not put the idea into the person's head. On the contrary, showing awareness of possible troubles and taking them seriously can open up much-needed lines of communication.
- STAY AS CALM AS POSSIBLE.
- DON'T INDUCE GUILT. Saying things like "You'll be throwing your life away," "It would hurt your parents so much," or "You've got so much to live for" may be counterproductive, raising a person's guilt or sense of hopelessness. Instead, focus on these facts: suicidal feelings are temporary, treatment exists, and people care.
- LISTEN. Encourage somebody who is suicidal to talk, and avoid arguing about or contradicting the content, even if it is illogical. Try to get a full picture of how the person sees the world; you can then better point out contradictions in his or her thoughts or judgments (such as how others will feel if they die) that the person may be denying or avoiding.

- SHOW YOU CARE. Say things like "I can tell you're really hurting" or "I care about you and will do my best to help you." Follow your words with action, such as helping the person find professional help or being attentive with visits or phone calls after the crisis has passed.
- GET HELP AS QUICKLY AS POSSIBLE. If the situation is acute, call 911 as soon as possible. If suicidal behavior is present but the threat is not immediate, seek a trained professional for help, and if possible, take the person at risk along with you. Suicide hot lines, a Samaritan center, family doctors or therapists, clergy members, or school counselors are all potential sources of help.
- DON'T LEAVE THE PERSON ALONE.

When a crisis passes, much work is usually required to rebuild tattered relationships, improve communication, foster insight and personal growth, and remedy problems (such as lack of parental attention) that contribute to suicide risk.

PREVENTING SUICIDE

Because many suicide attempts arise from untreated or inadequately treated major depressive disorder or bipolar disorder, identifying and treating these illnesses should be the first step in efforts to reduce suicide risk. As noted previously, the newer antidepressants appear to be particularly helpful in preventing suicide. Treating bipolar disorder with lithium has also been shown to significantly reduce suicide rates. In fact, as already noted, lithium appears to have specific antisuicidal effects for people with this disorder. Other psychiatric medications, including antipsychotics (especially Clozaril), also show promise for suicide reduction.[17]

Psychotherapy, particularly cognitive-behavioral approaches that include problem-solving training, reduce suicidal behavior more effectively than more reflective, or open-ended, therapies. Family therapy can be extremely helpful for troubled or suicidal teenagers. The goal in all cases is to correct and expand the constricted and warped thinking typical of suicide attempters, to open and improve communication, and to build psychological resilience, which, ultimately, is the best protection of all against the tragedy of suicide.

PART III

Anxiety and Depression
Among Women, Men,
Children, and Older Adults

10

ANXIETY AND DEPRESSION
IN WOMEN

My temperament, moods, and illness clearly and deeply affected the
relationships I had with others and the fabric of my work. But my
moods were themselves powerfully shaped by the same relationships
and work. The challenge was in learning to understand the complexity
of this mutual beholdenness and in learning to distinguish the roles of
lithium, will, and insight in getting well and leading a meaningful life.

— KAY REDFIELD JAMISON, PH.D., *An Unquiet Mind*

NEARLY TWICE AS MANY women as men are diagnosed each year with
either anxiety or depression. Women not only have some unique risk factors for the disorders, but they also experience some variations of anxiety
and depression specific to their sex. Women may encounter depression before menstruation, during pregnancy, and after the birth of babies. The differences in the quality and cycles of sex hormones between women and
men undoubtedly play some roles in these disorders, but many other factors also appear to be involved.[1]

- According to the 2002 *Summit on Women and Depression: Proceedings and Recommendations of the American Psychological Association,*
  women, more often than men, ground their self-concept on relationships. The frequent combination of sensitivity to relationship-based
  stressors and dependence on external validation of self-worth can lead
  women to become more upset than men over the distress of others
  and to neglect their own needs in an effort to please and serve others.
- Women tend to use a more ruminative way of coping, meaning a repetitive and introspective mental focus on distressing symptoms and
  their possible causes and consequences.

- Women are more likely than men to have been sexually or physically abused, which significantly raises one's risk factor for both anxiety and depression.
- Women are more susceptible than men to thyroid dysfunction, which influences mood.
- Women are more likely than men to admit feelings of depression and report past episodes of depression to physicians.
- Continuing inequality in wages and other forms of economic power, child care, housework, and ability to progress professionally can create stresses that exacerbate existing vulnerabilities to anxiety and depression.

In any given woman's life, factors such as these combine with the biological predispositions discussed in previous chapters to increase her vulnerability to an anxiety or depressive disorder. The degree to which these factors contribute to the roughly two-to-one disparity in the diagnosis of anxiety and depression remains unclear. In the 1970s, three women to every man sought professional help for depression, but a 2003 survey found that women outnumber men by only 1.7 to 1.[2]

ANXIETY AND DEPRESSION RELATED TO THE MENSTRUAL CYCLE

Compared with men, women experience tidal changes in levels of sex hormones such as estrogen, estradiol, progesterone, and follicle-stimulating hormone, all of which may affect mood and susceptibility to anxiety or depression. Such reproductive hormone fluctuations affect the hypothalamic-pituitary-adrenal (HPA) axis, which, as we have seen repeatedly, is a key player in how the body reacts to stress and how the mind responds with moods and emotions. (See Chapter 4 for more detail on the HPA axis.) Female hormone levels swing most widely during the menstrual cycle, pregnancy, and in the months or years leading to menopause.

Most women are aware of mood fluctuations before, during, or after menstruation. These are usually relatively mild and considered normal. When severe and debilitating, this is called premenstrual dysphoric disorder (PMDD), which affects from 3 to 8 percent of women, according to a 2003 report in the *New England Journal of Medicine*.[3] Women with PMDD suffer some combination of marked mood swings, depressed mood, irritability, and anxiety, which may be accompanied by physical symptoms such as appetite changes, lethargy, and sleep disturbances. The symptoms of PMDD closely resemble those of major depressive disorder or dysthymia. The key diagnostic difference is that symptoms are cyclic rather than constant and occur almost exclusively in the last two weeks of the menstrual cycle, just prior to menstruation. Unlike the effects of classic anxiety or depressive disorders, symptoms of PMDD usually disappear during pregnancy because of the cessation of menstruation. Women may experience premenstrual dysphoric disorder at any time during their reproductive years; its major physical symptoms are as follows:

- Headaches, migraines
- Abdominal cramps
- Bloating, weight gain
- Hot flashes
- Diarrhea, constipation
- General malaise, nausea
- Lack of appetite
- Skin changes, acne
- Heart palpitations
- Fatigue

Women suspected of having PMDD are usually asked to keep a careful record of their symptoms for two or more menstrual cycles. Women can also keep track of what they eat and drink, whether or how much they exercise, and major events in their lives as well as significant stressors. Such information can help a woman see the patterns of her symptoms and any relationships to potential triggers or exacerbating factors, such as excess caffeine consumption. To reduce the severity of symptoms of PMDD, women are encouraged to exercise and eat a healthful diet. Some studies show that daily doses of vitamin B_6 (50–100 milligrams) reduce the severity of depressive and physical symptoms.[4] Daily doses of 1,200 milligrams of calcium carbonate have also been shown to reduce physical symptoms such as water retention and food cravings as well as negative emotions.

If lifestyle and dietary changes do not adequately address symptoms, a physician may prescribe one of the newer antidepressants because in top-quality clinical trials such drugs have repeatedly been shown effective in treating PMDD. (For more detail about the newer generations of antidepressants, see Chapter 7.)

Antidepressants may be taken either continuously or only when symptoms appear. Several studies, including one from 2003, show that using antidepressants only when symptoms appear is more effective than continuous use.[5] Fortunately, the newer antidepressants usually relieve symptoms of PMDD within days, rather than the weeks required for relief of regular depression or anxiety.

But if a woman feels no response to an antidepressant after three menstrual cycles, other therapies can be considered, such as use of oral contraceptives or medicines that act on hormones, such as Lupron (leuprolide) and Suprefact (buserelin), both of which have been shown effective in good clinical research.[6] Although it was previously thought effective, research shows that the female sex hormone progesterone does not relieve symptoms of PMDD.

POSTPARTUM ANXIETY AND DEPRESSION

Childbirth is so cloaked with idealized imagery, expectation, and cultural symbolism that the sometimes difficult realities of this event can be easily ignored. Although childbirth and the first months of a newborn's life can be joyful and satisfying, they are also inevitably stressful, particularly for the mother. Sleep deprivation and the challenges of adapting to a new lifestyle can easily overwhelm new parents — even those with the blessings of an uncomplicated delivery, a healthy baby, intact and supportive families, and a stable home life.

Roughly three of every four new mothers, regardless of their circumstances, experience the "baby blues" — a period of sadness, irritability, anxiety, and confusion that typically peaks around the fourth day after delivery and resolves by the tenth day. For about one out of every eight new mothers, these symptoms linger and become the more severe and debilitating illness of postpartum depression (PPD).[7] The rapid changes in the levels of the female sex hormones estradiol and progesterone following childbirth have been implicated in PPD, though the exact mechanism of action remains unclear.[8] What *is* clear, however, is that women who have experienced a previous episode of depression are at higher risk for PPD. Here is the story of one woman who has described what she went through on the website of the Pacific Post Partum Support Society:

My early postpartum experience might best be described as subsisting. My daily goals included staying awake enough to feed and change my baby. Sleep deprivation became my number one enemy. I walked around hunched over like a ninety-year-old woman. With little or no sleep, I was shaky, weak, headachy, paranoid, irritable, teary, unmotivated, and I suffered blackouts upon rising too quickly.

In between my child's frequent cries for food, changing, and holding, I waited on pins and needles, knowing it would not be long until his next cry. Many calls to my husband at work, begging him to come home early or "right this minute," increased my self-loathing at being so helpless. Even when my child started sleeping through the night, my internal clock would not allow me to sleep, being trained to breastfeed every hour and a half by my infant's needy cries.

I bottomed out, wanting to just disappear with vague suicidal plans to just drive my car into a brick wall. I mistakenly believed everyone would be better off without me. I was desperate. Throughout this period, well-meaning family members would drop in to "help," expecting tea and sidestepping the colossal mess that once was an orderly house. They suggested getting up and exercising. I felt angry at their suggestions.

What I really needed was help with cleaning and child care while I slept. However, I didn't know how to ask for help yet, and they didn't know how to offer it. Somehow I kept going. It wasn't until the birth of my second child that I finally broke the silence about my postpartum depression with a good friend, who then confided that she too had suffered a mild PPD.

She gave me the phone number of a postpartum support organization. I was scared to call, but I was glad I did. I cried and cried on that first phone call and not once was I told to "get a hold of myself" or "just go to bed if you're sick." Instead I received reassurance — I was not going crazy, I deserved support, it was not my fault, and, best of all, things would get better.

Things have really changed for me now. I enjoy my children so much and have worked hard to maintain a balance between their needs and mine. I have learned that giving to myself is not selfish. When I nurture myself, I also nurture my family.[9]

Postpartum depression is serious both because of the suffering it causes the mother and the impact a dysfunctional mother can have on an infant. As discussed in Chapter 2, the ability of an infant to form strong bonds of attachment to caregivers (whether biological or adoptive) is important for later healthy development. Anxiety and depression interfere with the capacity to form such healthy attachments; hence, signs and symptoms of PPD should be addressed as quickly as possible.

Fortunately, PPD responds well to both psychotherapy (particularly interpersonal therapy) and medications — usually one of the newer antidepressants. In mild to moderate cases of PPD, it makes sense to try psychotherapy first, to avoid exposing a breastfeeding infant to antidepressant medications. (Depression After Delivery is a helpful nationwide advocacy group. For more information, see Appendix IV.)

If symptoms are severe, however, we believe that having an incapacitated mother poses more potential risk to an infant than does the relatively small risk involved in exposure to antidepressant medications. Unfortunately, doctors tell some women suffering from anxiety or depression that they must stop breastfeeding if they take an antidepressant or anti-anxiety medication. The many compelling advantages of breastfeeding outweigh the minimal risks involved with exposing an infant to an antidepressant via breast milk. To be cautious, however, most physicians advise that lactating mothers use the lowest effective dose. Prior to getting a prescription for an antidepressant, the mother should closely observe her infant's behavior so that fussiness or irritability is not later misinterpreted as a reaction to the mother's medication. Antidepressants are typically started at half the normal dose and continued for at least six months after full symptoms have disappeared, as a precaution against relapse.

The selective serotonin reuptake inhibitors Zoloft (sertraline) and Paxil (paroxetine) are recommended as first-line treatments for breastfeeding mothers because multiple studies suggest that they pose little risk due to their limited excretion into breast milk.[10] Studies of Luvox (fluvoxamine) also show no evidence of adverse effects on infants. But published reports suggest that Prozac may not be the best choice for lactating mothers. In one study, colic (continuous or excessive crying) was reported in three of the twenty-six infants who were breastfed by mothers taking Prozac, and these same infants gained significantly less weight than others did after birth, although the mothers did not report that the babies exhibited any unusual behavior.[11] Effexor (venlafaxine) is excreted into breast milk at relatively high concentrations, so this antidepressant, too, is probably best avoided by nursing mothers.

The older class of antidepressants, known as tricyclic antidepressants, is not typically found in measurable amounts in nursing infants, but these medications are seldom used these days. Children exposed to these medicines through breast milk have been followed through preschool and compared with children who were not exposed to such drugs, and no developmental differences have been found.[12]

Similar long-term evaluations have not been completed for infants exposed to SSRIs through breast milk. Research published in 2003 shows that peak levels of an antidepressant in breast milk occur eight to nine hours after ingestion, leading to the suggestion that mothers "pump and dump" breast milk at the eight-hour mark to minimize their infants' exposure to medications.[13]

Given how important it is for infants to have capable, supportive, and nurturing parents, it makes sense for women to strongly consider use of an antidepressant medication in conjunction with psychotherapy if they are depressed during any part of the pregnancy, postpartum, and breastfeeding phases of reproduction.

MENOPAUSE AND MOODS

The hormone changes of menopause do not directly cause either anxiety or depression.[14] Large-scale research studies have shown that most problems with depression begin when women are in their twenties or younger. It is actually unusual for depression to appear for the first time after menopause (defined as a year without menstruation).[15] Some studies, however, have found that during the months or years preceding menopause, women are somewhat more vulnerable to depression. The culprit may be the sleep deprivation caused by hot flashes and night sweats.[16] Insomnia can lead to irritability, fatigue, and increased vulnerability to a depressed mood. For some women — most notably those with a prior history of depression — these symptoms can progress to major depressive disorder. (For more information on depressive disorders, see Chapter 6.)

Nonbiological factors may also play a role. Perimenopause, the period before menopause, is often a time of changing roles related to retirement, children leaving the home, or responsibility for the care of ailing parents. Such transitions can elicit strong emotions such as feelings of loss, sadness, and uncertainty, all of which can trigger a preexisting vulnerability to anxiety or depression. Perimenopausal women who feel anxious or depressed should see their doctor for a complete physical examination to rule out other potential causes of the mood disorder. If no other explanations are found, a consultation with a psychiatrist or psychotherapist can be extremely helpful.

Optimal Treatment for Anxiety and Depression in Women

Though Chapters 5 and 7 provide guidelines for using psychotherapy and medications to treat anxiety and depression, a few issues specific to women must be added. For example, hormone replacement therapy (HRT) preparations are sometimes used to augment treatment with an antidepressant, even though the studies that support this pairing are old and their data are inconclusive.[17] This combination is even more problematic in light of studies published in 2002 and 2003, demonstrating that HRT does not confer some of the health benefits, such as protection from heart disease, that had formerly been claimed for it; also, it carries somewhat higher risks of inducing breast cancer than was previously thought.[18] Nonetheless, HRT usually relieves physical symptoms such as hot flashes, which sometimes improves mood because it promotes better sleep. And in a recent study of twenty depressed women being treated with estrogen alone, eight reported significant improvements in mood after eight weeks.[19] The authors of this small study note that larger placebo-controlled studies are required to confirm these results.

Ironically, depression is a rare side effect of HRT, for unknown reasons. (Some younger women who take birth control pills also report symptoms of depression.) When this happens to a woman who has never been depressed before, trying a different hormone preparation may help. However, women with significant histories of depression who become depressed again when starting HRT should switch to an antidepressant alone.

In all of these situations, a short-term course of psychotherapy should be tried in combination with the chosen medications. A treatment should be given adequate time to work before another is considered. A response to hormone treatment should occur within two to four weeks, whereas a full response to an antidepressant can take from six to eight weeks. If an antidepressant doesn't work in this time frame or produces intolerable side effects, a different medication should be tried; individuals vary widely in their reactions to these medications.

In addition to improving mood, SSRI antidepressants appear to have an added benefit for perimenopausal women. Recent research suggests that low doses of some antidepressants significantly reduce hot flashes and night sweats for some women. In a 2003 study, for example, women taking Paxil experienced half the number of hot flashes as did women taking a placebo.[20] This reduction is not as great as the 80 percent reduction typically seen among women who take hormone replacement therapy for hot flashes, but in light of the research mentioned earlier, many women now want to avoid the uncertainties of HRT, and thus Paxil or another SSRI might be a viable option for them.

Weighed against this potential benefit is the possibility of undesirable side effects from SSRI medications, such as weight gain and a reduced or delayed ability to achieve orgasm. It's difficult to predict whether a given woman will experience such side effects, though general information on the tendency of various antidepressants to exert these effects does exist. (See Chapter 7 for more detail on the common side effects of specific antidepressants.)

Women who experience weight gain or sexual side effects should talk with a psychiatrist or general physician. It is often possible to switch to another medication that produces fewer side effects but equal therapeutic benefit. Viagra (sildenafil) is often used to treat antidepressant-related sexual dysfunction in men, and some preliminary reports suggest it may increase arousal and ability to achieve orgasm in women as well.[21] Larger controlled trials to verify these findings are in progress, but women frustrated by this common side effect may want to explore this option with their physician.

Menstrual cycles, the hormone fluctuations of pregnancy and birth, and menopause can all contribute to the complicated biology of anxiety and mood disorders in women. Whether these unique aspects of womanhood account for the disparity between men and women in rates of diagnosis remains an open question. However, appreciating some of the unique factors reviewed here clearly makes it more likely that women struggling with anxiety or depression will get the support and treatment they deserve.

11

ANXIETY AND DEPRESSION
IN MEN

I was trying to buy happiness, and didn't understand the vicious cycle of depression. No one likes to admit there's something wrong — but you can get help. And you'll say, "God, why didn't I do this thirty years ago?"
— TERRY BRADSHAW, four-time Super Bowl champion quarterback[1]

"I DIDN'T WANT to get help," says Erik Elder (a pseudonym). "It was a macho thing."

Erik was trying to tough out a severe bout of depression — and he was losing. It was summer and for the previous six months he had had a nagging feeling that something was not right between his wife and his immediate supervisor at the company he worked for.

"Finally, on vacation with the kids, I overheard a conversation between him and my wife that confirmed everything I had been suspecting," he says. "The plan was to take my children and move out of state. That just tipped me over."

When it became clear his wife neither wanted to end the affair nor work on the marriage, he moved out.

"I was very, very depressed," he says. "I had two kids . . . a son who was seven or eight, and a daughter who was three or four years old. I couldn't sleep at night, so I took sleeping pills, but I just got less and less sleep and more and more depressed. Meanwhile I had to keep up with my job as a top executive of a large company."

Like many men, Erik plunged into work to distract himself from his pain. He says he didn't want to admit he needed help because, in part, he was afraid that if anybody knew he was having a psychological problem, his reputation as a leader in his industry would be ruined. But the pain was unrelenting.

"When you're as down and as low as I was . . . nobody wants to live like that," Erik says. "It's a living hell between your two ears. Worse than any physical pain you could have. It's totally debilitating. I used to hear that suicide is the ultimate act of selfishness because you don't realize the impact it has on other members of your family and the friends you leave behind. But people who have never been severely depressed don't know what it's like. It has nothing to do with leaving the ones you love. It has everything to do with stopping the pain. You simply cannot endure it anymore."

Finally, he took the advice of a close friend and sought help at a nearby hospital.

A doctor there tried three different medications before finding one that worked.

"I think I had been on the third medicine four to six days at that point . . . and the next morning I woke up and my attitude was decidedly different," he says. "For the first time my head felt somewhat light instead of heavy. It was unbelievable."

Erik's recovery also had a spiritual dimension he feels was as important as the medication. Although not a traditionally religious person, during the early days of treatment when nothing seemed to be working, he prayed for help. "I basically said, 'I've tried for five months to beat this thing, but I can't. I'm completely giving myself up to You.' It was powerful."

After his release from the hospital, he returned to his hometown and began the long process of divorce.

"Instead of getting sad, I was finally able to get mad at the situation and respond accordingly," he says.

Looking back now, he realizes that he had brief periods of melancholy prior to the discovery of his wife's affair and that other members of his immediate and extended family were touched with psychological problems. And although he wasn't enthusiastic about psychotherapy at first, Erik now says his many therapy sessions were key to his recovery.

"I think you need therapy to help you sort out what are normal thoughts and what are the negative thoughts generated by the depression," he says.

Erik eventually fell in love again, but before the wedding, he took his fiancée with him to a therapy session with his physicians so she could hear their perspective on his condition. He now lives with his second wife and the daughter from his first marriage. He still has occasional "slumps," but he says he knows now how to deal with them.

"Exercise is extremely important," he says. "It's a great tonic, not a cure-all, but it certainly helps with depression and I have found no substitute for it."

Erik is now CEO of a multi-million-dollar company. "Considering where I was, I feel like I've died and gone to heaven," he says. "I get about fourteen good days for every bad day. And I think there's still a lot of room for me to improve and to grow as an individual."

Overcoming the Hurdles

It will come as no surprise to most men (and women) that men consistently rank lower than women in their rates of consultation about anxiety and depression, in their willingness to confide their problems to others, and in acknowledging the need for help.[2] As Erik's story aptly illustrates, men sometimes delay seeking help until their condition reaches a crisis.

It's a hazardous pattern. Although roughly twice as many women as men are diagnosed each year with depression, men are four times more likely than women to commit suicide.[3] (Twice as many women as men are also diagnosed with the various anxiety disorders, with the exception of social anxiety disorder, which afflicts men and women equally.)

Men often experience depression differently from women and may have different ways of coping with the symptoms. For instance, men are more likely to acknowledge fatigue, irritability, loss of interest in work or hobbies, and sleep disturbances than feelings of sadness, worthlessness, and excessive guilt.[4]

Instead of acknowledging their feelings, asking for help, or seeking appropriate treatment, men may turn to alcohol or drugs when they are depressed, or they may become frustrated, discouraged, angry, irritable, and sometimes violently abusive. Some men, such as Erik, deal with depression by throwing themselves compulsively into their work, attempting to hide their condition from themselves, family, and friends; other men may engage in reckless behavior and put themselves in harm's way.

Men more often than women turn to alcohol and drugs when they are depressed, though in some cases the depression may arise from the substance abuse rather than vice versa.[5] Nevertheless, substance use can mask depression, making it harder to recognize depression as a separate illness that needs treatment.

Men may fail to seek help when they need it out of mistaken ideas about what psychotherapy entails. Perhaps surprisingly, many men still believe in myths about psychotherapy — that it involves lying on a couch to do free association, interpreting abstract inkblot patterns, or talking endlessly about one's mother. As we've explained, modern forms of psychotherapy, such as cognitive-behavioral, interpersonal, and family therapies, are quite structured, goal directed, and results oriented. Sessions focus on gaining insight into current problems and dysfunctional relationships rather than spending a lot of time reviewing the past. Of course, past personal history is often extremely relevant to current problems, and sometimes patterns of behavior or belief formed in childhood really do affect one's present state of mind. But clichés held by some men concerning the therapeutic experience simply don't exist in the real world.

Men battling anxiety or depression should also realize that they have company — roughly 12 million men suffer from depression each year, and millions more wrestle with anxiety disorders. Mental health professionals of all types are familiar with anxiety and depression in men, and any fears a man might have about admitting to a problem will quickly evaporate on the first visit. It is both wise and courageous for a man to seek help with problems. By seizing control of life in this way, he greatly increases the chances that he and his loved ones will be spared the misery and tragedy that so often accompany unacknowledged psychological illness.

RISK FACTORS

In addition to the general risk factors for anxiety and depression discussed in previous chapters, such as having a family history of either disorder and experiencing high and sustained levels of stress, certain risk factors are particularly pertinent to men.

- COMBAT EXPOSURE. Traumatic wartime experiences may predispose a person to later depression as well as anxiety disorders, particularly posttraumatic stress disorder. (Of course, this applies equally to women who have been in combat.)
- CHILD ABUSE. Although girls are more likely to be sexually abused than boys are, sexual abuse of boys does occur and can have devastating psychological consequences, in part because of the lingering

stigma surrounding homosexuality. In addition, boys often suffer more frequent or severe physical abuse than girls do.[6]

- JOB LOSS. Men tend to derive much more of their self-esteem from their jobs than women do; hence, the loss of a job, particularly one with high levels of prestige, power, or status, can precipitate anxiety or depression in men predisposed to these illnesses.
- DIVORCE. The stress and trauma of divorce hit men as hard as or harder than they do women.

ANXIETY, DEPRESSION, AND MALE SEXUALITY

Anxiety and depression can wreak havoc on the sex lives of both men and women, but far more research has been done about the impact on male sexuality. This may reflect a lingering stereotypical view that sex is more important to men than to women, the fact that most doctors and researchers are men, a real difference in the frequency of complaints between men and women patients, or some combination of these and other factors. Regardless of the cause for the unequal research, however, the results clearly demonstrate that anxiety and depression directly compromise erectile function and male sex drive.[7] The connection brings to mind the old joke about the brain being a man's largest sex organ. It's actually no laughing matter: sexual desire and a great deal of one's capacity to achieve and sustain an erection have everything to do with electrical and chemical activity in the brain. To the extent that anxiety and depression erode that activity, sexual performance suffers as well.

Psychological dysfunctions of many types can interfere with sex, and the mechanisms of the interactions are varied. For example, the relatively common phenomenon of "performance anxiety" among men begins with fearful anticipation of an erectile failure, which, in turn, activates the fight-or-flight anxiety circuitry detailed in Chapter 4. The combination of adrenaline release and activation of the autonomic nervous system makes it more difficult for the smooth muscles surrounding the arteries feeding the penis to relax and open up, which is the critical physical event behind an erection. Other types of physiological feedback loops are involved with depressive disorders, but the fundamental message remains the same: anxiety and depression block normal sexual response.

Of course, human sexuality is complicated, and many other factors can play a role in sexual problems. For instance, erectile dysfunction (formerly called impotence) is often rooted in physical problems such as diabetes-related nerve damage, cholesterol-clogged penile arteries, or the side effects of medication. Even if biology is initially to blame for erectile failure, however, the problem very quickly raises psychological issues — namely, performance anxiety, hesitancy to initiate sex, or withdrawal from a partner. Such reactions, in turn, can exacerbate the biological problems because the penis is a "use-it-or-lose-it" organ — reduced frequency of erections and/or orgasms can weaken penile tissues.

Anxiety and depression, therefore, can be both a cause and an effect of erectile dysfunction. Because roughly half of men between the ages of forty and seventy will experience some degree of erectile dysfunction at some point in their lives, this aspect of anxiety and depression affects millions of men.[8]

Treating anxiety or depression with psychotherapy, medications, or, preferably, both often improves erectile function and overall satisfaction with sex; however, it is also true that many of the most commonly used antidepressants actually *cause* erectile or orgasmic problems in men. Published studies suggest that from 30 to 60 percent of SSRI-treated patients may experience some form of treatment-induced sexual dysfunction, most commonly delayed ejaculation.[9] The wide variation in the reported incidence is due to differences in the definitions of sexual dysfunction used in the studies and also to the inherent difficulty of getting accurate information about a topic many men don't want to talk about.

Various strategies for the treatment of SSRI-related sexual dysfunction have been studied, including the following:

- Awaiting spontaneous remission of sexual dysfunction
- Reducing the dose of medication
- Taking a "drug holiday"
- Adding another drug to help reverse sexual symptoms
- Changing antidepressants
- Starting with an antidepressant known to have fewer or no sexual side effects

Wellbutrin, Serzone, and Remeron are the antidepressants currently on the market that produce the lowest incidence of sexual side effects.

Several studies, including one published in 2003, have demonstrated that some of the sexual dysfunction caused by SSRI antidepressants can be alleviated with Viagra (sildenafil)[10] or one of the newer erection enhancers such as Levitra (vardenafil). Other drugs, developed to treat Parkinson disease, such as Requip (ropinirole) or Mirapex (pramipexole), may also be effective in the treatment of SSRI-induced sexual dysfunction.

Another factor involved in both mood and male sexuality is the hormone testosterone. Medical research suggests that for men with below-normal levels of testosterone, boosting those levels slightly can improve mood, libido, and sexual functioning.[11] Social science research, on the other hand, demonstrates that higher-than-normal testosterone levels are associated with antisocial behavior, risk seeking, unemployment, and being unmarried, all of which raise the risk of depression. The effects of testosterone, in other words, are not nearly as simple as the media sometimes portray them, such as in advertisements for testosterone preparations aimed at men who want to build up their muscles.

Testosterone is not a valid general alternative to antidepressants or psychotherapy for depressed men. The research to date — and it has not been terribly thorough — shows that giving testosterone to depressed men with testosterone levels in the normal range has no antidepressant effect and may raise the risk for prostate cancer. Men with below-normal testosterone levels who have not responded to antidepressants, however, *have* been shown to respond positively to testosterone replacement therapy (delivered either with injections or a gel applied to the skin), according to a 2003 article by Harrison Pope Jr. and his colleagues at McLean Hospital.[12]

Interestingly, another 2003 study of older men found no differences in the mean testosterone levels between nondepressed and severely depressed men, but the older men with dysthymia (the chronic, low-grade form of depression described in Chapter 5) did have significantly lower testosterone levels.[13] It may be, therefore, that dysthymia is more directly linked to testosterone levels than major depressive disorder is.

Another line of evidence linking testosterone and depression comes from men being treated with testosterone-blocking hormones as part of prostate cancer treatment. One study found major depressive disorder in 13 percent of the men interviewed — roughly eight times the national average.[14] The risk was highest for men who had experienced a previous episode of depression.

Recent research has uncovered a link between high levels of

corticotropin-releasing hormone (which raises levels of the stress hormone cortisol) and testosterone. It appears that high levels of CRH reduce testosterone levels, which could exacerbate or initiate depression in vulnerable men. Whether the relationship between CRH and testosterone is reciprocal remains unanswered — we do not know, for instance, if raising testosterone levels reduces abnormally high levels of CRH.[15]

Research to date, therefore, suggests that the only valid application of testosterone is in the treatment of men with below-normal testosterone levels who have not responded to other medications. Even in this relatively small population of men, testosterone must be used very carefully because of its proven ability to promote the growth of prostate cancer. All men on testosterone replacement therapy should be monitored at least yearly — and preferably every six months — for levels of prostate-specific antigen (PSA), a marker for prostate cancer.

MEN AND DIVORCE

Contrary to the Hollywood cliché of the feckless man leaving his wife and children for another woman, divorce is more often initiated by women, and the psychological impact of divorce is harder, in general, on men.[16] In addition to higher rates of depression following divorce, divorced men are twice as likely to commit suicide as married men are, whereas no difference in suicide rates exists between married and divorced women.

The studies done to date suggest several reasons for men's apparent vulnerability to the psychological ravages of divorce. Women more often win full or majority custody of children, which for some men is a far more significant loss than loss of the spouse. As noted earlier, men also tend to deal with anxiety and depression in maladaptive ways, such as by using alcohol and drugs, becoming obsessed with work, or engaging in distracting activities. Women, on the other hand, tend to acknowledge and process their emotions by talking with others and relying on their social networks for help and support. Finally, men more often than women move out of the family home or apartment, which can be an isolating and destabilizing experience even when marital relations were tense or destructive.

Such facts should remind men and those around them to be particularly vigilant for signs of depression and anxiety in the months before, during, and after a divorce. Short-term, goal-directed psychotherapy can be invaluable during this time, as can appropriate medications if symptoms are severe.

The relationship between family problems and anxiety or depression is a two-way street. Clearly, an anxious or depressed man will be a more difficult partner and less effective parent. It is also true, however, that having a difficult spouse or troublesome relationships with children can exacerbate or cause anxiety or depression in men. These complicated psychological dynamics are often best addressed in family therapy, wherein some or all family members meet with a therapist to identify conflicts or difficulties, air feelings, and search for solutions and healing.

Unfortunately, men seldom initiate family therapy — or any therapy, for that matter. Wives or other female partners usually make the initial call seeking help and often spur men to attend therapy sessions. Whatever the reasons for this disparity in help-seeking behaviors, it remains an impediment to solving the very problems that bedevil so many men. The bottom line, as quarterback Terry Bradshaw has said, is that the sooner a man can accept that he needs help, the sooner he can regain control of his life and work toward greater psychological strength and resilience.

12

ANXIETY AND DEPRESSION IN CHILDREN AND TEENS

It is a wise father that knows his own child.

— WILLIAM SHAKESPEARE, *The Merchant of Venice*

THE FOLLOWING ARE POSTINGS from Teen Central, a website devoted to helping teens. They hint at the degree of angst, sadness, confusion, anxiety, and depression in the lives of many teens and young children today.

I hate my mom. I hate my life because it's so confusing. My girlfriend goes to a different school, and she's kind of acting mean so I might dump her. I like some other girl but I don't want my girlfriend to find out or she would freak out on me. I'm really confused, I don't know what to do. HELP ME!

I have nothing exciting to live for. I wake up, go to school, try my hardest, now starting tomorrow go to work, come home, do homework and sleep, over and over again. There is no one I can talk to. I feel so alone. I don't have great friends either. Everyone always creates a problem. I can't take this anymore.

Everything in my life is messed up. I moved out of my parents' house about three months ago, moved in with my close friend Jake, and since then everything has taken a turn for the worse.

. . . and she starts yelling for me to get off. I said, "No, I have nowhere else to lay down," and she slapped me in the face really hard. I was crying like crazy because this is the second time my mom has hit me. Does that sound like it is child abuse? Please help, I'm confused. Was that child abuse or verbal abuse? Emotional abuse maybe, because I'm really hurt.[1]

No Age Limit for Anxiety and Depression

Not until 1980 was an official diagnostic category created for childhood depression or anxiety. Until that time many clinicians assumed that young children, and even teens, didn't have the emotional or cognitive complexity to support true depression or anxiety. We now know this is false. Children as young as age two can become depressed, though their symptoms obviously take a different form from those of adults. One of every ten children and teens will suffer a mental illness severe enough to cause impairment.[2] Tragically, only about one fifth of these children get the treatment they need.[3] Tens of thousands of children, in other words, are falling through the cracks in family, school, and health-care systems. Childhood psychological problems not only cause needless suffering but also impair learning, disrupt relationships with family and friends, and can trap children in a downward spiral of dysfunctional behavior.

Detecting depression and anxiety in children and teens is difficult because their normal moods and emotions naturally swing more widely and less predictably than those of adults. It can be hard to know if a behavior pattern represents just a normal developmental phase or a sign of a disorder.

This chapter provides some guidelines for making such critical distinctions and for finding help if needed. The latest research shows that depression and anxiety in youth can be very effectively treated these days, though treatment methods must be tailored to the age of the child and differ in some significant ways from adult treatment. We'll look first at anxiety and depressive disorders other than bipolar disorder (BD) and then separately at BD. We will also discuss many practical ways to enhance resilience in children and teens, paying particular attention to the most widespread major stressor in children's lives: divorce.

Risk Factors in Childhood

As with adults, anxiety or depression seldom arises from a single factor, whether biological or related to life experience. The general rule presented in earlier chapters applies for young and old alike: inborn temperament and personality traits interact with life events and living situations to either increase or diminish a person's vulnerability to anxiety and depression.

That said, some important differences exist in the nature of the risk factors at work in young people.

As noted in Chapter 10, almost twice as many women as men are diagnosed with anxiety or depression. The situation is less clear for children, particularly preadolescents. Research suggests that more boys than girls are diagnosed with depression prior to adolescence.[4] Such figures must be taken with a grain of salt, however. Depressed preadolescent boys tend to become disruptive, fight with classmates and siblings, disobey teachers and parents, and break rules or laws. Such behavior attracts attention and raises the likelihood that the boy will be diagnosed. Depressed preadolescent girls, on the other hand, more often become quietly withdrawn, a less overt behavior and consistent with how many adults expect girls to act.

At puberty, rates of diagnosis reverse: twice as many teenage girls report depression, and their depressions tend to be more severe and longer-lasting than those suffered by boys.

Having closely related family members with anxiety or depression raises the risk for these ills in children. One study found that a young person who had one parent who suffered child or teen depression raised the chances thirteenfold that he or she would also experience early depression.[5] Studies of identical twins show that 30 to 40 percent of the time, if one twin suffers from anxiety or depression, the other will too. The rate for fraternal twins, who do not share identical genes, is from 15 to 20 percent. As with adults, therefore, genes play a role in vulnerability to anxiety and depression, but they do not rule. Many other factors combine to determine whether or not a vulnerability becomes an actual disorder.

Sadly, rates of physical, sexual, and emotional child abuse are high and climbing — though it is not known whether the actual rate is rising or whether more instances are being recognized and reported. Prevalence rates for child sexual abuse range from 12 to 35 percent for girls and 4 to 9 percent for boys, according to a study published in 2003.[6] The National Committee to Prevent Child Abuse estimates that roughly 3 million children are physically, sexually, or emotionally abused or neglected every year. Child abuse, therefore, is a very widespread risk factor for anxiety and depression in children and teens.

Of course, child abuse is also a risk factor for adult anxiety or depression. Studies show, for example, that women abused sexually as children are three to five times more likely to experience major depression or dysthymia as adults and have significantly higher risks for other mental disorders, such as posttraumatic stress disorder.[7] In a recent study of patients with chronic depression (lasting two years or longer), more than four of every ten subjects had been exposed to abuse, parental loss, or neglect during childhood.[8]

Another risk factor is unusual or sustained stress. Some stress, of course, is a normal part of growing up. Families move, friends leave, pets die, and peers can be cruel. But some children must cope with severe stress, and research shows this raises the risk that they will become anxious or depressed. The following life events prove to be the most profoundly disturbing for children of different ages, according to the widely used 100-point Coddington Scale of life stressors for children.

LIFE EVENT	PRESCHOOL	ELEMENTARY SCHOOL	HIGH SCHOOL
Unwed pregnancy	NA	95	92
Death of a parent	89	91	87
Divorce of parents	74	84	77
Marital separation of parents	74	78	69
Jail sentence of parent for more than one year	67	67	75
Becoming involved with alcohol or drugs	NA	61	76
Acquiring a visible deformity	52	69	81
Death of a sibling	59	68	68
Marriage of parent to stepparent	62	65	63
Hospitalization	59	62	58

NA = not applicable

Of course, these numbers should not be taken too literally. Different children will experience very different amounts of stress during an event such as a divorce, and this reflects their own resilience and the nature of the divorce itself. What matters most in any adverse event is the degree to which it disrupts a child's sense of security, attachment to parents and siblings, and sense of stability and safety, all of which provide the foundation for psychological health.

Having an anxious or depressed parent roughly doubles a child's risk for these disorders.[9] The influence is twofold: biological parents, of course, pass on some of their genes to their children, and equally important, a parent's ability to provide security, stability, affection, attention, and love is compromised by anxiety and depression.

The last significant risk factor is parental abuse of alcohol or drugs, which often leads to inconsistent or volatile behavior, neglect, and physical, emotional, or sexual abuse. In addition, parents' substance abuse often arises from an underlying mental disorder, which also raises the risk that children will suffer these ills.

GENERAL PRINCIPLES

Doctors can have a hard time figuring out what might be wrong with a child whose behavior is distressing to the child or those around him or her. Sometimes different doctors disagree about a diagnosis, or a parent may think that a given diagnosis doesn't fit what they observe day in and day out. These circumstances are, unfortunately, inevitable when dealing with emotional maladies in complex human beings. But even though diagnosis and treatment of children can be challenging, everyone involved should persevere because an effective treatment will likely be found eventually. The following guidelines may help in deciding how to deal with troubling behavior in a child or teen.

Trust Your Instincts

Parents generally know their children so intimately that they can detect even subtle changes in behavior and outlook. If you think something is wrong or different about your child, you're probably right — though, of course, that doesn't necessarily point to a serious problem. It is better, however, to make inquiries and be pleasantly surprised by the matter's benign origin than to assume it's "just a phase," only to be dismayed later by more radical and disturbing behavior changes.

Rule Out Physical Illness First

As with adults, the first thing parents or caregivers should do in response to a child's or a teen's troubling behavior is to schedule a thorough physical exam. As we have noted in previous chapters, many diseases and disorders create symptoms, such as tiredness or irritability, that can resemble signs of anxiety or depression.

Pay Attention to Children

This guideline may sound obvious, but particularly as children grow up and spend more time out of the home, it can be easy for busy parents to lose touch with their daily rhythms, habits, and behaviors. Only by paying close attention to these things will you notice the behavior changes that can signal distress. Of course, spending time with children, talking to them about their lives (even if they don't particularly want to), and paying attention to their concerns is not always easy or straightforward. It can require work to build enough trust and familiarity for children to open up about difficult or embarrassing aspects of their lives.

Deciding if a given behavior is worrisome or not depends critically on the context of the child's preexisting behavior patterns. Introverted behavior in a child who has always been vivacious or extroverted would raise concern, for example. In all cases, sudden changes of behavior in any direction should be addressed seriously. Behavior that changes subtly over the course of months or years is, of course, more difficult to spot and diagnose.

Deal Proactively with Your Own Anxiety or Depression

Parents with an anxiety or depressive disorder should learn as much as possible about the ways they might inadvertently foster such an illness in their children. Psychotherapy, either with or without children present, can be enormously helpful for learning ways to minimize harm to children and maximize their innate capacities to cope with stress or difficulties.

SPOTTING AN ANXIOUS CHILD OR TEEN

As in adults, anxiety disorders are the most common mental ills of childhood and adolescence. Researchers estimate that roughly one of every ten people age eighteen and younger experiences one of the following anxiety disorders:

- SOCIAL ANXIETY DISORDER. This disorder is characterized by extreme fear of embarrassment or being scrutinized by others. Children are sometimes diagnosed with a variant of social anxiety disorder called avoidant disorder, which involves a pervasive pattern of social inhibition, feelings of inadequacy, and hypersensitivity to negative evaluation.

- POSTTRAUMATIC STRESS DISORDER. This repeated reexperiencing of a traumatic event involves frightening, intrusive memories, hypervigilance, and deadening of normal emotions.
- GENERALIZED ANXIETY DISORDER. Sufferers experience persistent, exaggerated worry and tension over everyday events.
- PANIC DISORDER. In this disorder, extreme fear and dread strike unexpectedly and repeatedly for no apparent reason, often accompanied by intense physical symptoms such as chest pain, pounding heart, shortness of breath, dizziness, or abdominal distress.[10]

An additional anxiety disorder is specific to children: separation anxiety disorder, characterized by excessive anxiety surrounding separation from the home or adults to whom the child is attached. Symptoms of this disorder include:

- Extreme homesickness and misery when away from home
- Preoccupation with fears that accidents or illness will befall the attachment figures or themselves
- Reluctance or refusal to attend school or camp or to sleep over at friends' homes
- Inability to fall asleep without a parent or other attachment figure present
- Nightmares
- Physical complaints (stomachaches, headaches, nausea) upon separation

Anxiety disorders are as disabling for children and teens as they are for adults. Relationships fray, schoolwork suffers, health declines, and self-esteem sinks. If left untreated, anxious children will likely grow into anxious or depressed adults. A study published in 2001 found that adolescent anxiety, particularly social anxiety disorder, strongly predicts depression later in life, which is another indication of how intimately bound together these two disorders are.[11]

To some extent, anxious children are simply born that way. Research by Harvard psychologist Jerome Kagan and colleagues clearly demonstrates that even as infants, children display distinct behavior patterns that predict later anxiety. Kagan finds that up to one of every five children is irritable as an infant, shy and fearful as a toddler, and cautious, quiet, and introverted upon reaching school age. He calls such children "behaviorally inhibited." (This is not a diagnosis of a disorder but rather a characterization of the more introverted end of the normal spectrum of personality traits.) In contrast, as many as one third of infants are bold, gregarious, and unperturbed by novelty — they are behaviorally uninhibited. The remaining 50 percent fall somewhere in between.[12]

Kagan has shown that behaviorally inhibited children display a characteristic set of physical responses when exposed to unfamiliar events; these responses closely mirror the types of physical symptoms displayed by anxious adults. Inhibited children, for example, show faster heart rates, higher blood pressure, and less heart-rate variability than noninhibited children do in unfamiliar situations. Kagan suggests that the inhibited children have a more highly reactive central nervous system in general, and in particular greater sensitivity and reactivity in their hypothalamic-pituitary-adrenal (HPA) circuit, as do adults with an anxiety disorder.[13] (For more information on the HPA axis and anxiety in general, see Chapter 4.) Work by Kagan and others shows that inhibition remains relatively stable over time and that early inhibition correlates strongly with later anxiety disorders.

Anxiety disorders in children and teens tend to "co-travel" with other disorders or problems, such as substance abuse, attention deficit/hyperactivity disorder (ADHD), and conduct disorders such as oppositional-defiant disorder. It can be difficult to determine whether the anxiety disorder is the root disorder or if other disorders are primary because each exacerbates the others. Overt, disruptive behavior garners the attention of parents and teachers and thus may appear to be the primary problem when, in fact, an underlying anxiety or depressive disorder is at work.

Determining if a child's anxious behavior qualifies as a true anxiety disorder may not be a straightforward process. It can be easy to forget what it's like to be a child or teen; children's anxiety can seem, to adults, to be out of proportion to a prospective event. Going to school for the first time, a first date, performances, and athletic events can all trigger considerable anxiety in children and teens, and these normal responses should not be mistaken for an anxiety disorder. Again, the key things to watch for are anxious behaviors that persist for more than two weeks, sudden behavior changes, or anxiety that interferes with schoolwork, relationships, or daily life. In such cases, trust your instincts, and take your child to a professional for a proper diagnosis.

SPOTTING DEPRESSION

When confronted with a typical loss, such as the death of a grandparent or pet, or an upsetting or frightening situation (changing schools, moving, being bullied, and so on), children can feel real grief, sadness, or rage. They may complain of body aches and pains, have bad dreams or trouble sleeping, experience changes in appetite, or regress behaviorally. Such reactions are normal and typically abate within days or, at most, a week or so. However, experiencing a major life stressor, such as an act of terrorism or the death of a parent, will elicit longer-lasting and more severe emotions and moods.

Thus, determining if a child's behavior and symptoms qualify as signs of true depression requires consideration of both the symptoms themselves and the context in which they occur. Here are the major signs for children who aren't yet teens:

- Easily aroused frustration, irritability, or volatile mood (unusually violent play, bullying, angry outbursts, and so on)
- Loss of interest in formerly enjoyable activities (suddenly considered "dumb" or "boring")
- Significant weight loss or gain
- Frequent unexplained stomachaches, headaches, or bodily pain
- Altered sleep patterns or sudden requests to sleep in a parent's bed
- Fatigue, lack of energy
- Frequent sadness, feelings of worthlessness, or inappropriate guilt
- Sudden problems with paying attention or concentration
- Recurrent thoughts of death or suicide

A child must display five of these symptoms most of the time for at least two weeks to be formally diagnosed with depression. Don't wait to intervene, of course, if a child displays fewer but severe symptoms. When in doubt, always seek professional help — starting with the child's pediatrician or family doctor.

The signs of depression — along with practically everything else —

change when children move through puberty, a time that can sometimes stress out even the most well-balanced adolescent living with the most loving, supportive, and stable family. Adapting to emerging sexuality, peer pressure, parental expectations, and the need to establish an independent identity can result in depressive, anxious, or disruptive behaviors. Because adolescents typically shift their confiding relationships from their parents to their peers, parents can feel cut off, rejected, or out of touch even when they make strenuous efforts to connect. Faced with a belligerent, stubborn, or overtly hostile teen, parents can easily become fed up and, even if they don't say so explicitly, give up trying to communicate.

When diagnosing depression in teens, psychiatrists use the same basic set of symptoms listed earlier for diagnosing depression in children, though the symptoms often take different forms:

- Self-destructive behaviors (having unprotected sex, abusing alcohol and other drugs, or obsessively picking at or irritating parts of the body)
- Eating-related difficulties, particularly for girls (sudden changes in appetite, binge eating, or excessive dieting)
- Sudden social isolation
- Extreme sensitivity to rejection or failure
- Sudden change in physical activity (either becoming lethargic though normally energetic or restless and agitated though normally placid)
- Morbid or unusually intense interest in death or suicide

If a teenager displays some of these symptoms or some others listed previously, try to probe what's going on by talking with him or her. If you are repeatedly rebuffed or become so frustrated that you feel like giving up, seek professional help — a family doctor, adult or child psychiatrist, or family therapist, for example. The grim statistics on the pervasiveness of teen psychological illness cited at the beginning of this chapter suggest that far from being overcautious, many parents are not taking action as soon or as effectively as they could.

OPTIMAL TREATMENT FOR ANXIETY AND DEPRESSION IN CHILDREN AND TEENS

With proper treatment almost all childhood anxiety or depressive disorders can be overcome. As with adults, the basic therapeutic options are psychotherapy, medication, or a combination of the two for more serious problems. As a rule of thumb, we suggest trying psychotherapy before medications unless a child or teen is obviously suicidal or posing a danger to self or others. Try to identify and begin to address any life circumstances that might be contributing to an anxious or depressed mood, such as conflicts with peers, parents, or teachers; fears or uncertainties about sex; difficult home or school transitions; difficulty with meeting parental expectations; or inadequate nutrition and exercise. Psychotherapy can often be extremely helpful in these efforts — and can help whether or not a child or teen attends the sessions — because in therapy, parents often learn valuable new strategies and approaches for dealing with their children.

Finding solutions and getting optimal treatment depend critically on proper diagnosis. If a physical exam rules out thyroid dysfunction, mononucleosis, and other potential physical causes of depressive or anxiety symptoms, a child or adolescent should be evaluated by a child psychiatrist or other trained specialist. This usually involves taking a thorough family history, talking with parents and the child or teen, and asking a series of questions directed to either the parent or child as appropriate, the answers to which are recorded, given numerical scores, and then summed to gauge the severity of the situation. Many scales of depression or the various anxiety disorders have been specifically tailored for use with children of different ages, and these scales have been rigorously tested for their reliability in detecting or predicting a mood or anxiety disorder.

If a child or teen is acutely suicidal, dependent on alcohol or another drug, manic, or so functionally impaired that daily activities are disrupted, hospitalization should be very seriously considered. If suicide is even a remote possibility, parents should remove from the house any potentially hazardous medications, guns, knives of all sorts, or other potentially dangerous substances or objects. The odds that potentially suicidal adolescents will kill themselves double when a gun is kept in the home, according to a 2003 study.[14]

Psychotherapy

Regardless of the severity of symptoms, we believe psychotherapy should be a standard part of any treatment program for children and teens with anxiety or depression. Children and teens have much to learn about themselves, the disorder, and how to cope with difficulties in their lives, and therapy can be an excellent forum for such discoveries. Cognitive-behavioral therapy and interpersonal therapy are the most rigorously studied psychotherapies among populations of depressed or anxious children and teens; as noted by David Brent and Boris Birmaher in the *New England Journal of Medicine* in 2002, most studies show that these techniques are roughly as effective as medications.[15]

In cognitive-behavioral therapy young people learn to increase pleasurable activities, improve interpersonal effectiveness, and identify and modify dysfunctional and self-defeating patterns of thought that can lead to depressed mood. In interpersonal therapy, children and teens learn to cope with relationship difficulties (such as loss of a boyfriend or girlfriend) and manage their transition to independence. The language and techniques used in therapy vary with the age of the patient. Young children or children with limited verbal sophistication will often be asked to draw or use dolls to express feelings or explore troubling situations in their lives. Older or verbally adept children can interact with a therapist as adults do, though the therapist will tailor the vocabulary, analogies, and explanations to the level of the child or teen.

However, some adolescents are extremely resistant to traditional forms of psychotherapy — meaning one-on-one dialogue between the therapist and the adolescent, which takes place in a room or office. In such cases, a more physically active type of therapy may help, such as art therapy, drama therapy, music therapy, outdoor wilderness experiences, or participation in activities on a working farm or ranch. Another possibility is involvement in programs that match teens with trained peers or that group peers to work on similar challenges.

Traditional psychotherapy for children typically involves eight to sixteen weekly sessions, though more or less frequent sessions may be warranted. Even after symptoms have abated and stability has been restored, therapy is often continued on a monthly basis for an additional six months to decrease the risk of relapse.[16]

In cases of suicidal behavior, some studies find that creating a "no-suicide pact" between a depressed child or teen and parents or a clinician reduces the risk of suicide.[17] The patient agrees to contact a responsible adult (not necessarily a parent) or the therapist if he or she feels suicidal. If developed with the full participation of the child or teen (rather than being thrust upon the person), a no-suicide pact can strengthen relationships and clarify issues that may underlie suicidal behavior.

Family therapy, in which some or all family members participate in sessions, can be extremely helpful in cases of child or teen anxiety or depression. Sharing information, explanations, and feelings among all affected parties minimizes miscommunication or misperception of important issues. Family dynamics that might have contributed to a disorder can reveal themselves when relevant family members are present, which can be valuable for all.

Finally, relaxation training can help some adolescents. Usually offered by psychotherapists specializing in anxiety disorders, this instruction helps people differentiate states of arousal and tension from a state of relaxation, detect early signs of becoming tense, change behavior before a spiral of anxiety sets in, and learn specific relaxation techniques, principally deep breathing and systematic muscle relaxation.

Medications

Most parents are understandably cautious about treating their child's psychological illness with medications — and, generally, the younger the child, the more cautious the parent. This is a prudent approach because we still lack definitive answers to some key questions:

- How effective are antidepressants and anti-anxiety medications for children and adolescents?
- What are the long-term effects of antidepressants or anti-anxiety medications in children?
- Do developing brains respond differently to medications than adult brains?
- Will medications used in youth affect the need for medications in adulthood?

Until we can answer such questions definitively, it makes sense to be conservative with medications. That means trying nonpharmacological treatments first and weighing the known benefits of medications against the risks of *not* treating a disorder with medications. In general, the more serious the condition, the more strongly a trial with a medication should be considered.

Short-term studies show that some of the selective serotonin reuptake inhibitor (SSRI) antidepressants, detailed in Chapter 6, relieve anxiety in children and teens. The most compelling studies indicate that Prozac (fluoxetine) and Luvox (fluvoxamine) are effective for child and adolescent anxiety. Emerging data suggest that Paxil (paroxetine) and Zoloft (sertraline) are similarly effective.

The situation differs for children and adolescents with depression. Controlled clinical trials show that Prozac[18] and possibly Zoloft[19] can relieve depression in children and teens. But no such evidence exists for Paxil and Effexor (venlafaxine). Whether these latter antidepressants are truly less effective in children and/or adolescents is unclear because nearly as many study participants responded to the placebo as the antidepressants, which makes it hard to demonstrate the efficacy of any drug.

Of considerable concern, however, are data from the makers of Paxil and Effexor indicating increases in mood instability and thoughts of suicide in a small number of depressed children and adolescents treated with these agents. These increases were greater than those seen in children who received a placebo. As of early 2004, the most prudent approach is to avoid these two medications as first-line treatments of depression in children or adolescents. At that time, an advisory panel to the FDA recommended adding a warning about the possibility of increased suicidal behavior in children and teens to the labels of all SSRIs.[20]

These notes of caution should not be misinterpreted. Much compelling evidence suggests that SSRI antidepressants in general *reduce* suicide risk and that failing to treat adequately children or teens at risk for suicide or severe depression will do more harm than good.[21] No actual suicides were reported in any study — only increases in suicidal ideation. Many questions remain; more research should clarify the matter.

And as noted, these medications *have* been shown effective in conditions other than depression for this age group — for example, social anxiety disorder — and many practitioners believe that these drugs are effective for young people. If a patient at any age receives benefit from a given medication and has had no significant side effects, we would recommend that the treatment continue. Note, however, that little evidence exists to suggest that the older tricyclic antidepressants are effective in children or adolescents and these drugs have cardiovascular side effects of particular concern in this age group.

As we've mentioned, antidepressants take time to kick in, usually at least two weeks for the start of a therapeutic effect and then up to eight weeks for a complete effect. This lag time should be clearly explained to children and teens, who might otherwise expect the kind of fast response they have experienced with painkillers. Whether they are sexually active or not, teenagers should also learn that all SSRIs can interfere with sexual functioning by impairing erectile function or delaying or dampening orgasm. Because teens tend to be very concerned about sexuality, they should also be assured that other medications can be tried if the one they are currently taking causes undesirable side effects.

Although antidepressants are usually the first-choice drugs for anxiety disorders these days, the benzodiazepine medications such as Xanax (alprazolam) and Valium (diazepam) can alleviate some anxiety symptoms and are commonly used for all anxiety disorders except posttraumatic stress disorder. (For more detail about these drugs, see Chapter 5.) The potential for abuse of benzodiazepines is relatively low, though teens with a history of substance abuse should avoid the stronger and faster-acting benzodiazepines such as Halcion (triazolam). At low doses, benzodiazepines can be used in the long term without fear that larger and larger doses will be required. However, teens need to understand that benzodiazepines amplify the sedative effects of alcohol and barbiturates, making the combination hazardous.

The doses of all medications are modified for young children to account for lower body weight and metabolic differences. Medications are typically begun at a fraction of the normal adult starting dose, taken for a week, and then raised to a weight-adjusted full dose if no unacceptable side effects occur. Further adjustments in dose may be required because children and teens often metabolize medications more rapidly than adults do; thus, higher doses than might be expected are sometimes needed to achieve optimal treatment. In one study, for example, more than seven of every ten young patients who had no response to the typical 20-milligram adult dose of Prozac (fluoxetine) showed pronounced improvement on higher doses (40 to 60 milligrams).[22]

Many medications have not been officially approved by the FDA for children because drug companies have not conducted the requisite controlled clinical trials. This does not mean such medications should not, or cannot, be used (with the exceptions noted previously). Physicians may prescribe medications for conditions or patients not specifically mentioned in the formal FDA approval paperwork, a practice called off-label prescribing, an extremely common, accepted component of modern medicine.

Physicians generally prescribe off-label when preliminary clinical reports from other physicians suggest a medication will be safe and effective for a new population or for a new type of disorder.

When a medication is FDA-approved for children, the age given on the label should not be viewed as a rule, but rather a guide, because the age limit is driven by the design of the clinical trials that preceded approval, not by evidence that the drug is either dangerous or ineffective at younger ages. For example, the stimulant Ritalin (methylphenidate) is formally approved for children age six and older because the studies on which the approval was based involved children age six and above. But this doesn't mean the drug is unsafe or ineffective for younger children.

SPOTTING AND TREATING CHILDREN AND TEENS WITH BIPOLAR DISORDER

As we described in Chapter 8, bipolar disorder and its less severe form, cyclothymic disorder, arise from malfunctions in the brain circuitry controlling the swings and cycles of emotion. The normal highs of pleasure, joy, and contentment and the normal lows of sadness, grief, and disappointment become exaggerated and prolonged. Contrary to previous notions, recent studies show that bipolar disorders are as common among youth as among adults.[23]

These disorders are wrenchingly difficult for both the suffering young person and, almost always, for the parents or guardians. To say it is "challenging" to parent a young person with bipolar disorder is to engage in woeful understatement. Here, for example, is Maya's experience ("Maya" is a pseudonym).

> For the first nine or ten years of my daughter's life, we thought that we just had a strong-willed child. She would be a little difficult to manage, but not horrible, just like a regular child, no violent behaviors or anything. Then we moved after living in the same place since my daughter was two.
>
> Leaving her close friends was difficult. About a week before we moved, she screamed at me when I asked her something. When I told her one night to take her bath, she refused and got very angry. When I pursued the request, she came into the living room, picked up a clock,

and threw it across the room, which scared the hell out of me. I had never seen this.

In the weeks following the move, she was miserable. After she started her new school, I started getting phone calls two or three times a week with problems. The kids would say something to her, she would get mad, and then she would cry, which made her even madder. Then she started having these "episodes" at home, starting at about one or two a month, lasting thirty to forty-five minutes. If I asked her to do something she didn't want to, she became very angry and eventually violent. She would punch me, kick me, and say horrible things right to my face. Then I noticed how her face would change. I would try not to cry, but I always did, and she would get in my face and laugh, and I swear she looked like a demon. She looked as if she would kill me. After a few minutes, her face would totally change and the tears would come.

These episodes became more frequent and lasted longer, so we went to counseling and a psychiatrist, who put her on medication for ADHD, which did nothing. I kept looking for help. One night we had a major blowout. My husband had to hold her off me and literally sit on her, to keep her from coming at me. She was extremely verbally and physically abusive. We called the hospital I'd been talking with and was told to call 911, which I did. Later that night, we were in a psychiatric hospital. A wonderful doctor took her case, heard about my family history, and correctly diagnosed her with bipolar disorder.

My daughter was started on medication, and after three weeks, she was a changed person. She still has her moments and has had the medication adjusted a couple of times, but she is about 85 percent better than she was. She's an A/B student, smart as a whip, and involved with good people, friends, and church.

As a mother, I personally know what it's like to have your life turned upside down. If we could have diagnosed her a little sooner, it would have been great. I was afraid one of us would kill the other. Even though she's much better, she still can have outbursts, which are painful to me. Being a mom of a child with bipolar disorder can be especially tough. It helps to know there are others out there.

Maya's story illustrates the severity of the mood changes typical of bipolar disorder. Her daughter's behavior was far more extreme than the moodiness and irritability common among adolescents. On the other hand, Maya's daughter is a classic "good responder" to medication, and not all young people respond as quickly or as thoroughly as she did. Finding the right medication, or combination of medications, can be tricky and time-consuming. In addition, entrenched psychological dynamics in the patient and his or her family take time to change and evolve to more satisfying and productive patterns. Experts cannot yet predict which medication will work best for a given patient with bipolar disorder, nor can they predict which side effects a child or teen will experience. Children, teens, and their caregivers need perseverance and patience as they move through the process of diagnosis and treatment.

The symptoms of bipolar disorder in children and teens differ in some important ways from symptoms typical of adults. When manic, for instance, children and adolescents tend to be irritable and prone to destructive outbursts rather than feeling elated or euphoric, as is common for adults. When depressed, children and teens tend to complain of the same constellation of symptoms discussed earlier: headaches, stomachaches, tiredness, sudden behavior changes, irritability, unexplained or frequent crying, social isolation, poor communication, and extreme sensitivity to rejection or failure.

More often in children and adolescents than in adults, mania and depression occur as "mixed states": the irritability or erratic temper of mania blends with the moody, bleak outlook of depression, or manic and depressive periods cycle unusually rapidly — over a period of days or even hours.[24]

Research published in 2003 suggests that the presence of a manic episode is the clearest sign of pediatric bipolar disorder — and that such mania can be differentiated from the superficially similar extroversion of attention deficit/hyperactivity disorder (ADHD).[25] The mania of bipolar disorder is more extreme and frequent, and it lasts longer than the giddiness of healthy children or the excitability or "hyper" behavior of children with ADHD. In addition, for children with bipolar disorder, switches into mania involve more than just mood: such children usually experience a decreased need for sleep, grandiose ideas, increased goal-directed activity, heightened sexuality, and increased pleasure seeking. That said, the line between bipolar disorder and ADHD is blurry, and many — perhaps most — children with bipolar disorder also exhibit signs and symptoms of ADHD.

Studies suggest that bipolar disorder beginning in childhood or early adolescence may be a different, possibly more severe form of the illness than the type that emerges during older adolescence or adulthood.[26] When the illness begins before or soon after puberty, it is often characterized by a continuous, rapid-cycling, irritable, mixed-symptom state that may co-occur with disruptive behavior disorders. In contrast, onset of bipolar disorder in later adolescence or adulthood tends to begin suddenly, often with a classic manic episode, and to have a more episodic pattern, with relatively stable periods between episodes.

A child or adolescent who appears to be depressed or to have very high energy for more than two weeks, or who exhibits severe symptoms with excessive temper outbursts and mood changes, should be evaluated by a psychiatrist or psychologist with experience in bipolar disorder, particularly if a family history of the illness exists. This evaluation is especially important because stimulant medications such as Ritalin (methylphenidate, often prescribed for ADHD) and SSRI antidepressants may trigger or worsen manic symptoms.

Because a biological dysfunction clearly lies at the root of bipolar disorder — more so than for either anxiety or depression — newly diagnosed individuals should almost always be immediately treated with both medications and psychotherapy. Little research has as yet been conducted on the efficacy and safety of using mood-stabilizing medications in youth; hence, treatment approaches are based mainly on experience with adults.[27]

The medications used to treat bipolar disorder vary with the stage of the illness. Acute mania, for example, requires a fast-acting drug such as one of the benzodiazepines or one of the atypical antipsychotics, for example, Zyprexa (olanzapine), Geodon (ziprasidone), or Risperdal (risperidone). Once the mania has subsided, however, lithium or one of the other mood-stabilizing drugs is appropriate. Possible side effects such as acne or weight gain may be particularly important to monitor for at this age. Note that valproic acid (sold under various trade names, such as Valproate and Depakote), a common mood stabilizer for adults, may not be preferred for young women. Studies conducted in Finland show that this drug may increase testosterone levels in teenage girls, which can disrupt menstruation, promote weight gain, and induce abnormal hair growth.[28] Several large studies funded by the National Institute of Mental Health are now examining the value of long-term treatment with lithium and other mood stabilizers in preventing recurrence of bipolar disorder in adolescents. These studies will also assess side effects and overall adherence to treatment.

The depressive phase of bipolar disorder is sometimes treated with an antidepressant, though this must be done cautiously because antidepressants can sometimes induce mania. Clinicians need to use great care in taking a history in cases of childhood or adolescent depression because signs of mania may not have appeared yet or may have been too mild for parents to recognize them for what they were. In the absence of such clues it's impossible to tell if a given case of child or adolescent depression arises from bipolar disorder or a depressive disorder that does not involve elevated moods; hence, close attention is needed during the early weeks of treatment with an antidepressant. (For more information about antidepressants and other medications for bipolar disorder, see Chapter 8.)

Regardless of the medication used, bear in mind these points:

- Like adults, teens are sometimes tempted to stop taking their medication because they miss the "highs" of mania. Children and teens should not be left to take their medications on their own — drugs should be kept in a safe place and dispensed by the parent.
- Both parents and young patients should understand that bipolar disorder, like other chronic disorders such as diabetes, usually requires taking medication indefinitely.
- Alcohol and other recreational drugs reduce the effectiveness of medications for bipolar disorder and should be avoided.
- Parents play a critical role in monitoring a child's compliance with taking medications and working to heal and understand usually complex emotional dynamics.

COPING WITH TRAUMA

Since September 11, 2001, almost all parents in the United States have had to grapple, to one degree or another, with how best to help their children understand horrific, terrifying events. Most parents now have dealt with a situation that used to afflict only those who suffered more personal or limited traumas, such as the death of parents or family members, serious accidents, or a natural disaster.

We hope the following suggestions will not have to be implemented on as wide a scale as needed in the weeks after September 11, but given the unavoidable uncertainties of life, it is prudent for parents to prepare themselves with this type of information.

Both adults and children who experience catastrophic events vary in their responses, depending, in general, on their level of resilience. Some suffer only worries and bad memories that fade with emotional support and the passage of time. Others are more deeply affected and experience long-term problems that require professional help. Emotional reactions such as fear, depression, withdrawal, or anger can occur immediately after a tragic event or weeks or months later. Loss of trust in adults and fear of a recurrence of the event are common among children and adolescents after such a cataclysm, though other reactions vary with age. Children younger than age five may display fear of being separated from a parent, crying, immobility, aimless activity, trembling, or excessive clinging. They may also regress to earlier behaviors such as thumb sucking, bed-wetting, and fear of darkness. Older children may show extreme withdrawal, disruptive behavior, or inability to pay attention. Also common are physical complaints, avoidance of school, decline in academic performance, sleep disturbances, and confusion.

Bear in mind the following suggestions for helping children or teens cope with tragedy:

- Explain the episode of violence or disaster as well as you can, in language and detail appropriate for the age or sophistication of the children.
- Encourage children to express their feelings and listen to others without passing judgment. Help younger children find the words to describe their experience. However, do not force them to discuss the traumatic event.
- Let children and adolescents know it is normal to feel upset after something bad happens.
- Allow time for youngsters to experience and talk about their feelings. At home, however, a gradual return to routine can be reassuring.
- If children are fearful, reassure them that you and others love them and will take care of them. Stay together as a family as much as possible.
- If behavior at bedtime is a problem, give children extra time and reassurance. Let them sleep with a light on or in your room for a limited time, if necessary.

- Reassure children and adolescents that the traumatic event was not their fault.
- Do not criticize regressive behavior or shame a child with words like *babyish.*
- Allow children to cry or be sad. Don't expect them to be brave or tough.
- Encourage children and adolescents to feel in control by letting them make some decisions about meals, what to wear, and so on.
- Find time to take care of your own needs so you can better take care of the children.[29]

THE SPECIAL CASE OF DIVORCE

National tragedies, such as the attacks of September 11, and personal tragedies, such as the death of a parent, are certainly stressful and can cause intense emotional turmoil for children and adolescents. But these events are not the only and certainly not the most common cause of major childhood stress. As noted earlier, the divorce of a child's parents ranks number three in terms of psychological impact (see page 168). Because divorce is so common these days, it warrants special attention for anyone who cares about anxiety and depression in children and teens.

Parents sometimes erroneously think that because divorce is so common, it is also a "normal" experience for children. It is not normal, but rather a world-overturning event, and it takes months for a child to fully recover from it. A divorce does not, however, need to be catastrophic or leave lasting psychological scars. Unlike the death of loved ones or terrorism, some aspects of a divorce can be controlled. Parents can transform an unavoidably painful and difficult transition into an experience from which both they and their children can emerge with greater psychological health and resilience. Here are some suggestions for achieving this desirable — if difficult — goal.

Be honest about the implications of the divorce. Don't pretend the transition will be easy or painless. Acknowledge that divorce is serious and painful for everybody involved but that, in the opinion of at least one parent, the existing situation is even worse. Be prepared to answer the same questions repeatedly — young children, in particular, may understand something intellectually but not really grasp its full impact or be able to connect emotionally until something concrete happens, such as the absence of a parent from the dinner table.

Try to see things from your children's perspective. Where you may see relief, freedom, or opportunity, they may see only loss, change, and uncertainty. Children and teens are invariably frightened and confused by divorce because it threatens their security — even when the existing situation is untenable because of abuse or neglect. Reassure children that the divorce was not their fault (a common belief), that you still love them deeply, and that you will help them in the weeks and months to come, no matter what.

Pay attention to signs of unexpressed feelings. If a child says he or she is "fine" but acts distinctly "not fine," bring it up and ask questions. Be prepared for wide swings of emotion, from grief and intense sadness to anger and outright hostility. Look also for behavior changes such as those that signal either anxiety or depression (as discussed previously).

Give children and teens plenty of advance warning about impending changes, such as a move or a parent's departure from the home. Talking about it and allowing them to process the information and emotions over a period of days will minimize the trauma and allow them to feel more in control of the situation.

Maintain daily structure and routines as much as possible by, for example, keeping children in the same child-care centers or schools, sticking to normal meals and bedtimes, maintaining consistent limits on inappropriate behavior, and continuing contact with familiar friends or family members. The more structure and security you can build into children's lives, the better they will cope with the upheaval.

Make every effort to avoid criticizing, insulting, or demeaning the other parent in front of the children. This self-discipline can be astonishingly difficult in the midst of rejection, betrayal, abuse, grief, or manipulation. When in the midst of intense emotions, try to avoid talking about the other parent until feelings have cooled.

Avoid turning a child into a confidant or a "miniature adult." Don't ask children to assume responsibilities beyond their abilities, such as requesting that a six-year-old make his or her lunch every day or assigning a teen to arrange child care for a younger sibling. Although children and teens may be eager to help, they deserve to remain children and teens, not adults.

Move slowly with new relationships. Children need time to adjust to a divorce — and the younger the child, in general, the more time it takes. Introducing a new relationship adds stress and uncertainty to a child's world; hence, it's better to give a child time to adjust to one change (divorce) before making another. New partners should be slowly integrated into the home and family.

Seek support groups, friendships, and counseling. Single parenting is hard work, particularly if, as is common these days, extended family members live too far away to help out. Reaching out to clergy, friends, relatives, and groups such as Parents Without Partners can help both parents and children adjust to the travails of separation and divorce (see Appendix IV for contact information).

RAISING RESILIENT CHILDREN

Dealing with a child or a teen with an anxiety or depressive disorder involves more than diagnosis and treatment. These are young people, after all, and their personal and social development is anything but finished. Caring adults can take positive steps to help a youngster move beyond the level of physical and mental health that existed prior to an illness and raise his or her resilience for facing future bouts of anxiety or depression. Building this quality is an ongoing process. The unavoidable stresses, pain, and disappointments of life can be treated as opportunities to teach children to master and respond appropriately to emotional pain.

As discussed in more detail in Chapter 2, stressful events that are followed by rest and recovery time can build resilience, whereas continuous stress (such as that caused by ongoing abuse) fosters anxiety and depression. Be alert to stressful moments, and try to provide rest, security, and "time off" to allow a child or teen that invaluable recovery period.

The first step in fostering resilience is to accurately assess a child's temperament and typical behavior patterns. This task is not as trivial as it may sound. Many parents or caregivers naturally want their children to behave in certain ways or respond to events just as they would respond. Although perfectly normal, this tendency can result in conflict when a child is simply not the person a parent wants him or her to be. Intellectual parents, for example, may want their children to excel in academic subjects, and they become frustrated if the kids show no interest in such matters. Normally quiet, reserved parents can be baffled or irritated by an expansive, exuberant, "feisty" child.

In such cases parents need to step back from their desires and expectations and try to see who their children really are. Are they inhibited or outgoing? What really makes them happy? What kinds of things do they do when left on their own? The answers to such questions are the foundation for interactions that promote self-esteem and mastery.

Knowing and accepting a child's personality do not mean accepting all behaviors or becoming a passive parent. All children need structure, high expectations, and clear rules for behavior. The child who is not athletically inclined still needs to exercise and might gain a great deal by being encouraged to participate in a team sport. Likewise, the creative, artistically inclined teen still has to master high school math and language arts, even if those skills don't come naturally. The goal is not to eliminate all stress but to avoid protracted stress caused by a mismatch between what a parent or caregiver wants and what a child or teen is really cut out for.

Building resilience requires a foundation of consistent, predictable expectations and rules at home. If two parents are involved in child rearing, they should try to agree on rules for behavior and work out their own differences away from the children. (This applies equally when custody is split and the parents don't live together.) Familiar routines and rituals, such as making family dinner a priority even when work demands or after-school activities make it difficult, contribute to fostering a sense of stability. Standard bedtimes and going-to-sleep routines can help as well and may include reading together, listening to music, or, for younger children, singing prior to bedtime.

Part of being resilient is having a realistic view of the world — and that includes the bad or painful parts of it. In general, children benefit more from the truth than from half-truths or "white lies" spoken in the mistaken belief that a child "can't take it." Simple, straightforward responses tailored to the age of the child are the best way to deal with questions about death, sex, drugs, catastrophic world events, or other sensitive subjects. This approach lets children know they can handle the truth, which in turn bolsters their confidence (in addition to giving them vital information, of course). A related issue is allowing children to engage with the world even when this entails some risk. As we noted in Chapter 2, exposure to situations that mimic a real stressful or dangerous event toughens a person's psychological and physiological responses. Letting young people engage in sports or activities that entail some risk of disappointment or injury engages this process in relatively controlled and safe surroundings.

Contact sports such as soccer or basketball, outdoor activities such as skateboarding or skiing, and family activities such as hiking or bike riding all provide opportunities for teaching children that they can survive both physical and emotional slings and arrows. (Obviously, reasonable safeguards such as helmets, pads, or trained instruction should be used when appropriate.) An important secondary benefit of these types of activities is physical exercise, which itself is an important prerequisite to resilience.

These are challenging times to be a parent — and challenging for children and teens as well, particularly if they are vulnerable to anxiety or depression. Fortunately, proven, effective treatments exist to help such children. All parents — whether their children struggle with a disorder or not — can take relatively simple steps with their children every day to lay the foundation for their well-being as adults.

13

ANXIETY AND DEPRESSION
IN OLDER ADULTS

> To resist the frigidity of old age one must combine the body, the mind,
> and the heart — and to keep them in parallel vigor one must exercise,
> study, and love.
>
> — KARL VON BONSTETTEN, author, 1745–1832

AT EIGHTY-SIX, Dora Bakish walks and talks with a refined authority. Fluent in several languages, an impeccable dresser, and unfailingly polite, she divides her time between a home in Montreal and one on the French Riviera.[1] This is a far cry from the condition in which Bakish had found herself three years ago. Then she was sitting alone on a freezing balcony, shivering in her nightdress, unable to move or to breathe normally. Only a call to 911 kept her from succumbing to hypothermia.

"I had this feeling in here that's indescribable," she told a reporter with the *Toronto Globe and Mail* in 2002, clutching her hands over her heart. "It wasn't sadness, it was anxiety . . . overwhelming anguish in my soul."

In the previous weeks, her energy had melted away. Overwhelmed by daily living, she did nothing. Her weight dropped to 94 pounds from her usual 118. After more than eight decades as a whirling dervish, she became, in her words, "a log."

Dora was suffering from both anxiety and depression. Yet when she arrived at the emergency room after coming down from the balcony, she was prescribed sleeping pills and sent home.

"They pegged my mother as another sad old lady," says David Bakish, her son, who is a psychiatrist. "With older people, they tend to do that; they say, 'She's getting older, of course she's depressed.' But I don't think depression is any more normal for an eighty-three-year-old than for a twenty-three-year-old."

David was deeply concerned by his mother's mood changes and continued to press her to seek help. He finally convinced her to admit herself to the Royal Ottawa Hospital, which specializes in geriatric psychiatry. She spent months in treatment as the doctors searched for the right combination of psychotherapy and medication. She is now taking Effexor XR (venlafaxine) as well as Aricept (donepezil hydrochloride), a drug used to treat the early symptoms of Alzheimer disease.

"Ultimately, my son saved my life because he got me help," Dora says.

Dora's anxiety and depression dissipated. She returned home and got back to her normal weight and her busy social calendar.

"At eighty-six, I am not a young woman, but getting treated has made me feel a lot younger," she says. "My story should tell everyone that you should not abandon people because they are old. Our problems, our depression, can be resolved."

Not a Normal Part of Aging

Dora was lucky. Far too often, both physicians and family members overlook older adults' symptoms of anxiety or depression; the same symptoms would, however, trigger concern or alarm if observed in younger people. The infirmities, losses, and aggravations of age can make anxiety and depression seem like rational responses rather than the pathological, potentially life-threatening diseases they really are.

Generally speaking, anxiety and depression strike up to one of every ten people who are older than age sixty-five. Certain groups of older adults, however, have higher rates of depression. As many as one in five nursing-home residents is clinically depressed.[2] Those percentages translate into staggering numbers: from 2 to 5 million older adults in the United States alone suffer from depression, and millions more battle anxiety.[3]

These mental diseases take a tragic toll, not just in suffering, but in lives. Older Americans are disproportionately likely to die by suicide. Comprising only 13 percent of the U.S. population, individuals age sixty-five and older accounted for 18 percent of all suicide deaths in 2000.[4] Particularly vulnerable are white males age eighty-five and older, whose suicide rate is five times the national average. Tragically, several studies have found that up to three quarters of older adults who killed themselves had visited a primary-care physician within a month of the suicide, which illustrates both the difficulty of diagnosis and the pressing need for physicians to practice heightened vigilance in detecting signs of anxiety or depression in the elderly.

Some patients and physicians remain stubbornly mired in misunderstanding about anxiety and depression. A survey by the National Mental Health Association found that more than half the older adults polled thought that depression was a normal part of aging, and half thought depression was a "personal weakness."[5] Nothing could be further from the truth.

It's true that older adults experience more loss, discomfort, pain, and disability than younger people do. Faced with such difficulties, it is normal for older adults to experience short-term anxiety, grief, sadness, irritability, or any of a number of other emotional reactions (just as younger people do when they face difficulties). But anxiety and depressive disorders are, by definition, abnormally protracted and severe versions of normal moods that should be taken seriously and treated as quickly as possible.

Treating the anxiety and depression of older adults can be more complicated than similar treatment for younger people, and the disorders are sometimes more difficult to diagnose. But the costs of misdiagnosis and undertreatment greatly outweigh the challenges posed by these disorders. Many studies prove that treatments effective for the young are equally effective for the old.[6] Psychotherapy, medications, electroconvulsive therapy, or a combination of these treatments can almost always alleviate symptoms and restore normal functioning. Treating the anxiety or depression, in turn, enhances recovery from other illnesses and can free older adults to engage in the kinds of healthful practices that bolster resilience and make further episodes of anxiety or depression less likely.

BARRIERS TO DIAGNOSIS

Anxiety and depression can be more difficult to detect in older adults for the following reasons:

- Older adults sometimes don't recognize their own symptoms, believing they are a normal part of aging.
- A desire to avoid being a burden to others or appearing weak and vulnerable sometimes leads older adults to consciously or unconsciously

deny their feelings to family and physicians — a phenomenon some-times called "masked depression." They sometimes put on a happy face during meetings but revert to feeling miserable when alone.

■ Older adults suffer more physical ills, such as uncontrolled diabetes, heart disease, osteoporosis, stroke, and cancer, all of which can pro-duce symptoms that distract attention from co-occurring anxiety or depression.

■ Some common medications, or the interactions of medications, can produce side effects such as agitation or lethargy, which mimic symp-toms of anxiety or depression.

■ The aging process itself can complicate the interpretation of symp-toms. Certain physical symptoms such as changes in appetite and sleep patterns as well as fatigue are recognized as signs of depression in younger adults. But older people who are not depressed often expe-rience such changes as a natural part of aging.

■ Older adults are less likely than younger people to complain of sad-ness, hopelessness, or feelings of worthlessness, focusing instead on physical aches and pains or other problems such as difficulty sleeping and fatigue. This pattern is another form of "depression without de-pression" or "masked depression."[7]

That said, the sets of symptoms used to diagnose anxiety or depres-sion, discussed in Chapters 4 and 6, apply to older adults as well. The same general rules apply too: symptoms must be persistent (most of the day, nearly every day, for at least two weeks) and severe (they must interfere with daily functioning and life activities).

ANXIETY AND DEPRESSION OCCURRING WITH OTHER ILLNESSES

As discussed in Chapter 3, depression often co-occurs with other serious illnesses, such as heart disease, stroke, diabetes, cancer, and Parkinson or Alzheimer disease. In such cases, health-care professionals may mistakenly conclude that mood changes or alterations in bodily function are due to the chronic illness. This dynamic contributes to the underdiagnosis and undertreatment of anxiety and depression in older people.

Additionally, these disorders often co-occur with substance-abuse disorders in older adults. Alcohol or drug dependence can exacerbate existing anxiety and depression, and they can also create anxiety and depression, either via a direct biological action or as a result of withdrawal symptoms when a substance is unavailable (such as when a patient enters a hospital or nursing home). Substance use must be discontinued in order to clarify the diagnosis and maximize the effectiveness of psychiatric interventions. Additional treatment is necessary if the depression or anxiety remains after the substance use and withdrawal effects have ended. Individuals or family members with concerns about the co-occurrence of anxiety or depression with another illness should discuss these issues with a physician.

Some symptoms of depression occur as a factor of other medical conditions. For example, weight loss, sleep disturbance, and low energy can accompany diabetes and heart disease; apathy, poor concentration, and memory loss are also found in Parkinson and Alzheimer diseases; and achy feelings or fatigue may characterize many other conditions. To determine the proper diagnosis, a physician must conduct a thorough evaluation, keeping in mind that depressed older people are more likely to complain of physical problems than to express sad, anxious, or hopeless feelings.

IS IT DEPRESSION OR DEMENTIA?

One illness can be particularly difficult to distinguish from depression: dementia (a common form is caused by Alzheimer disease). Forgetfulness, confusion, and chronic irritability are symptoms of both depression and dementia. When an underlying depression causes symptoms similar to those of dementia, a patient is said to have depressive pseudodementia. Because the symptoms of pseudodementia are rooted in depression, memory problems and confusion can disappear with proper treatment. At first glance dementia and pseudodementia look similar, but a closer look reveals distinct differences.[8] Here are several symptoms of pseudodementia:

- Onset can be dated with some precision.
- Rapid progression of symptoms occurs after onset.
- Patients usually complain much of cognitive loss.
- Complaints are usually detailed.
- Patients usually communicate a strong sense of distress.
- Cognitive dysfunction is stable from day to night.

- "Don't know" answers are typical in response to questions probing cognitive function.
- Memory loss for recent and remote events is usually equally severe.
- Loss of social skills often occurs early and is prominent.

Roughly 2.3 million people in the United States have been diagnosed with Alzheimer disease, with another 360,000 cases reported each year.[9] About 3 percent of men and women ages sixty-five to seventy-four have the disease, with incidence increasing with age beyond that. It now appears that in addition to memory lapses, mild confusion, and disorientation, a depressive disorder is also one of the earliest symptoms that may appear. Psychiatric disturbances of some kind occur in about nine of every ten Alzheimer victims, with depression and anxiety being the most common.

The natural history of depression in Alzheimer disease is still poorly understood, but the association between the two highlights the importance of getting prompt diagnosis and treatment. Depression and agitation, two of the most common symptoms of Alzheimer disease, in turn worsen nearly every aspect of the disease. Studies show that depressed Alzheimer patients have a higher risk for disability in activities of daily living, physical aggression, being discharged from an assisted-living facility, entry into a nursing home, suicide, and death.

Interestingly, the depression and anxiety seen in Alzheimer victims don't appear to be reactions to the knowledge and burden of having the disease, but to brain damage at the root of the memory, cognitive, and physical disabilities. Research published in 2003 suggests that experiencing depression earlier in life raises one's risk of getting Alzheimer disease.[10] This seems to be true even when symptoms of depression occurred more than two decades before a diagnosis of Alzheimer disease. The reason for this link is unknown, but the findings may indicate that the disease starts earlier in life and manifests itself in subtle ways around middle age. Alternatively, early-life depression may in some as-yet-unknown way lower a person's neurological resilience, leaving him or her more vulnerable to the physiological deterioration of Alzheimer disease.

How best to treat anxiety and depression in Alzheimer patients is still unclear. Studies of antidepressant medications have produced contradictory results — some showing benefit, some not. Psychotherapy for patients and caregivers does not appear to reduce immediate symptoms, though it may improve secondary aspects of the disease, such as relationships between family members.[11]

Here are the current recommendations for treating anxiety or depression in those with Alzheimer disease:

- Provide psychotherapy for both the patient and primary caregiver (unless symptoms are severe; see end of list). If the patient does not respond within eight weeks of psychotherapy, antidepressant medication (typically an SSRI) should be considered.
- Develop clear daily routines, and arrange for pleasant activities for the patient.
- Educate caregivers about dementia and depression.
- Assess the problem-solving skills and physical capabilities of the caregiver so assistance can be provided if needed.
- Initiate antidepressant medication or electroconvulsive therapy if symptoms include suicidal or violent behavior or if the patient is not eating or drinking adequately. (See Chapter 7 for more information about antidepressants and ECT.)

BARRIERS TO TREATMENT

Some formidable barriers make it difficult for some older adults to get the help they need. For example, as noted earlier, a powerful stigma about mental illness still exists among older adults, many of whom may have grown up with the notion that experiencing anxiety or depression denotes a "weak character"; strong people simply "pull themselves up by their bootstraps." Psychological difficulties also threaten independence, which is something many older adults are both proud of and scared of losing. Such thinking interferes with making accurate judgments about the extent and severity of one's difficulties; it also blocks the normal impulse to reach out for help and support.

Some older adults are hampered by lack of money or accessibility. Even those who are insured may not have coverage for psychotherapy, or their prescription coverage may entail such high copayments that medications are prohibitively expensive. Many older adults take multiple medications, which can add up to a significant monthly expense. Finally, many older patients cannot drive or have difficulty using public transportation.

The sheer effort or hassle of getting to and from appointments can be so daunting that an older adult will simply give up.

OPTIMAL TREATMENT FOR ANXIETY AND DEPRESSION IN OLDER ADULTS

Both antidepressant medications and short-term psychotherapies, particularly cognitive-behavioral therapy and interpersonal therapy, can effectively treat late-life depression. Psychotherapy alone has been shown to prolong depression-free periods of good health, though combining psychotherapy with medication usually provides maximum benefit.[12] In one study, about four of every five older adults who received combination treatment recovered from depression.[13] Combination treatment was also found to be more effective than either treatment alone in reducing recurrences of depression.

The selective serotonin reuptake inhibitor (SSRI) family of antidepressants is usually considered the first-line medication choice for treating both anxiety and depression in older adults. Older medications, including tricyclic antidepressants and monoamine oxidase inhibitors, however, also effectively relieve depression, and some people respond better to these drugs. The generally higher incidence of troublesome side effects with these medications, especially low blood pressure that causes fainting, makes them less than ideal for older patients, however. (For more detail about antianxiety medications, see Chapter 5; for information about antidepressants, see Chapter 7.)

Choosing among the many medications available for anxiety and depression is complicated for older adults because of the following factors:

- Older adults often metabolize drugs more slowly than younger people do, leading to higher-than-expected levels of the drug in the blood. Some physicians thus sometimes adopt a "start low, go slow" approach to drug prescription, though other physicians prefer a more aggressive approach, starting with normal doses and increasing rapidly if no therapeutic effect is seen.
- Many older adults already take drugs for medical conditions such as high cholesterol, high blood pressure, and pain. Some of these drugs can adversely interact with certain antidepressants because they are metabolized by the same enzymes in the liver. (See Appendix III.)

- Older adults tend to be more sensitive to side effects related to heart function, such as rapid heartbeat, low blood pressure, or high blood pressure.

As we've already mentioned, many new antidepressants and anti-anxiety medications are in development, and these hold particular promise for older adults because, in general, they appear to produce fewer side effects and have less impact on the cardiovascular system than current medications do. The clinical trials conducted to date have not involved enough older adults to warrant firm conclusions, but preliminary results are promising.

Electroconvulsive therapy is also a viable option for older adults and has been proved as safe and effective for this population as for younger people, though some older patients experience longer-lasting memory and cognitive impairment following ECT, the severity of which tends to increase with the patient's age.[14] ECT can be particularly appropriate for patients already using a number of medications, for whom adding yet another medication is inadvisable.

PREVENTING DEPRESSION, CULTIVATING RESILIENCE

As Mae West once said, "You're never too old to be younger" — younger, anyway, in terms of psychological and physical resilience. Whether or not a person has been diagnosed with anxiety or depression, he or she can work toward greater resilience and reduced vulnerability to these and other mental ills. For more background and details about resilience in general, see Chapter 3. Here are some specific ways older adults can increase their resilience.

- MAKE CONNECTIONS. Get involved in civic groups, faith-based organizations, or other local groups. Another way to connect to others is to offer help in times of need even if you can contribute only in a small way.
- ACCEPT CHANGE AS A PART OF LIFE. Coming to terms with circumstances that can't be changed helps a person focus on areas of life where he or she can make a positive difference.
- TAKE SMALL STEPS TOWARD A GOAL. Ask, "What's one thing I can accomplish today that helps me move in the direction I want?"
- LOOK AT THE BIG PICTURE. Stressful or emotionally wrenching

experiences can narrow a person's focus, making life seem hopeless or overwhelming. Find ways to regain a broader, long-term perspective. Some people find that meditation, yoga, exercise, or getting involved with young people can help with this.

■ TAKE CARE OF YOURSELF. Psychological resilience is rooted in physical resilience. Try to exercise regularly, eat healthful foods, and engage in pleasant, relaxing, or stimulating activities.

These suggestions should be tailored to fit your own lifestyle, values, and abilities. And they don't need to be accomplished overnight. Make small changes, and take one day at a time.

As Bette Davis noted, "Old age is no place for sissies." She's right — aging often brings new and sometimes very difficult challenges related to physical and circumstantial changes, which sometimes lie largely beyond one's control. But anxiety and depression are not among those inevitable changes. These two afflictions of the mind and body are never normal at any age. No older adult should suffer from anxiety and depression in this day when so many effective treatments exist. And we are not simply talking about medications. Visits from caring relatives, attention to little needs or concerns, and help with mundane aspects of daily living are as important as maintaining proper neurotransmitter levels to a resilient, positive outlook on life.

APPENDIX I

COMPLEMENTARY AND ALTERNATIVE MEDICINE

Complementary and alternative medicines include medical and health-care systems, practices, and products not presently considered part of conventional medicine. Some practices, such as acupuncture, have been proved safe and effective for certain applications and are being adopted into conventional health care. But many techniques have not yet been studied scientifically. This doesn't mean they might not have value; it just means that we, as medical scientists, cannot recommend such techniques without reservations.

Complementary medicine techniques are used together with conventional medicine. For example, yoga or meditation can be practiced at the same time a patient is receiving conventional treatment for anxiety. Most physicians and mental health workers view complementary therapies positively because they may enhance recovery and pose very little risk. However, before engaging in a complementary technique (particularly one that involves aerobic activity), patients should check with their physician for advice concerning any limits that might be appropriate for their particular level of health and condition.

Alternative medicine practices are used in place of conventional medicine. For example, a person may use a special diet to treat anxiety or depression rather than psychotherapy or medications recommended by a conventional doctor. We know that some people harbor deep distrust of the medical "establishment," and, indeed, we acknowledge that conventional medicine is hardly perfect. Our bias, however, favors what is known as evidence-based medicine. Although obtaining evidence is usually difficult, time-consuming, and expensive and is never 100 percent accurate, we believe history demonstrates that this approach works better than using treatments based on hearsay, studies of very small numbers of people, or studies so seriously flawed in their methods as to render their results meaningless.

We urge anyone interested in pursuing an alternative therapy to talk to his or her doctor about it beforehand. An M.D. may know valuable information, such as new findings about potentially harmful interactions between herbal products and other medications. In addition, while a person is engaged in an alternative therapy, a disease such as anxiety or depression may worsen. People owe it to themselves to cover their bases as best they can, even if they believe strongly in an alternative approach. And in the end, the final decision belongs to the patient, for he or she will live with the consequences.

Medical workers need to recognize that four of every ten American adults use at least one type of alternative therapy every year. Physicians and mental health workers should educate themselves about the range of products, techniques, and therapies used outside of their practices and be willing to constructively engage with patients so that health and well-being can be most optimally achieved.

Both complementary and alternative techniques have been classified in five broad categories by the National Center for Complementary and Alternative Medicine, an arm of the National Institutes of Health. They are alternative medical systems, mind-body interventions, biologically based therapies, manipulative and body-based methods, and energy therapies.

ALTERNATIVE MEDICAL SYSTEMS

Alternative medical systems build on systems of theory and practice that have evolved apart from and earlier than the conventional medical approach used in the United States. Examples include homeopathic medicine and naturopathic medicine. Examples of systems that have developed in non-Western cultures include traditional Chinese medicine and Ayurveda.

MIND-BODY INTERVENTIONS

Mind-body medicine uses a variety of techniques designed to enhance the mind's capacity to affect bodily function and symptoms. Some techniques that were considered alternative in the past have become mainstream (for example, patient support groups and cognitive-behavioral therapy). Other mind-body techniques are currently considered complementary, such as meditation, prayer, mental imaging, and therapies that use creative outlets such as art, music, or dance.

BIOLOGICALLY BASED THERAPIES

Biologically based therapies use substances found in nature, such as herbs, foods, and vitamins. Some examples include dietary supplements, herbal products, and the use of other so-called natural but as yet scientifically unproven therapies (for example, shark cartilage to treat cancer). For a thorough discussion of the herb most widely used to treat depression, Saint John's wort, see Chapter 7.

MANIPULATIVE AND BODY-BASED METHODS

Manipulative and body-based methods are based on manipulation and/or movement of one or more parts of the body. Some examples include chiropractic or osteopathic manipulation and massage.

ENERGY THERAPIES

Energy therapies involve the use of alleged energy fields. Biofield therapies are intended to affect energy fields that purportedly surround and penetrate the human body. The existence of such fields has not yet been scientifically proven. Some forms of energy therapy manipulate biofields by applying pressure and/or manipulating the body by placing the hands in, or through, these fields. Examples include qi gong, reiki, and therapeutic touch. Bioelectromagnetic-based therapies involve the unconventional use of electromagnetic fields, such as pulsed fields, magnetic fields, or alternating current or direct current fields.

Appendix II

Making Sense of
Health Information

All statements or claims in this book are backed as fully as possible by evidence from research studies published in journals after peer review. Since other forms of media also discuss the issues of anxiety and depression, we want to offer basic information that will help you evaluate the strength of health-related claims.

Physicians and researchers sort available information on any topic into three broad categories called levels of evidence. The highest level consists of either randomized, controlled clinical trials or high-quality reviews of other studies (meta-analyses). In randomized clinical trials, participants are assigned to receive either a treatment of some kind (a drug, for example), or a placebo (dummy pill). The choice is usually made by using a computer program that simulates a random event, such as the flip of a coin. Usually, neither the participants nor the people conducting the study know which subjects are getting the real treatment and which are getting the placebo — a situation called a double-blind trial. If both the research doctor and trial participants know which medication is being used, the trial is called open-label.

Such "blinding" of researchers and participants reduces the chance that a person's expectation about a treatment will bias his or her observations — a phenomenon called the placebo effect. The placebo effect is particularly strong in studies of antidepressants and anti-anxiety medications. It is not uncommon for up to 40 percent of participants getting a placebo in such trials to report feeling less depressed or less anxious.

After a specified amount of time, the outcomes in the two groups of a randomized clinical trial are compared. Some studies include rules for stopping a trial early if either significant negative effects are found or such positive effects are found that it is unethical to continue denying the treatment to all study participants.

The other type of study that generates the highest level of evidence is called a meta-analysis, which compares and contrasts a set of previously published studies. The results are summed up in an attempt to discern patterns underlying studies of the same basic phenomenon. A meta-analysis, of course, is only as good as the studies on which it is based, but this approach is an invaluable tool for synthesizing information from many researchers over the course of years. For example, the 1996 review by Klaus Linde and his colleagues of research on the effectiveness of Saint John's wort for treating depression, mentioned in Chapter 7, is a meta-analysis.

Midlevel evidence is provided by observational studies in which large groups of people are tracked, often for years. Observational studies are the only way scientists can ethically address questions such as whether people with Alzheimer disease have a history of depression, or whether those with panic attacks tend to consume more caffeine than average. When researchers start to analyze the information from an observational study, they try to be sure the groups they are comparing are equivalent — a process called controlling for variables. For example, some people who consume large amounts of alcohol also smoke cigarettes. Before valid conclusions could be drawn about the health of heavy drinkers compared with nondrinkers, the smokers in the alcohol-drinking group would have to be removed from the analysis.

The fundamental drawback of observational studies is that people choose their treatments or behaviors, and those who drink heavily, take vitamin pills, or exercise, for example, may differ in fundamental ways (such as their genetic makeup) from those who do not. This phenomenon is called "responder bias," and it can exert a significant, and often invisible, influence on results. For example, several large, well-designed observational studies found that women who took hormone replacement therapy at menopause had a reduced risk of having heart attacks. But when careful randomized clinical trials were conducted to prove this finding, no difference was found. The discrepancy probably lay in the fact that women who chose to have HRT were, by and large, thinner, healthier, and wealthier than the women who did not choose HRT, and it was these differences, not the HRT, that caused the differences in heart attack risk. When the differences were avoided with randomization, the effect disappeared.

The lowest level of evidence comes from so-called expert opinion or consensus viewpoints, which are often formalized summations from a group of experts. The opinions and beliefs of clinicians play a vital role in directing future research efforts and, at times, bringing to light important new discoveries. For example, in 1953, physician David Bosworth noticed that the patients who were getting a new drug for tuberculosis seemed remarkably happy for people who had holes in their lungs. His observations, picked up by Nathan Kline, set the wheels in motion for development of one of the first monoamine oxidase inhibitor antidepressants: iproniazid.

Sometimes the only available evidence is expert opinion — for example, when a medication has not been rigorously tested in children. In such cases, parents and their child's physician must rely on the clinical experience of other physicians, both published and word of mouth, in making treatment decisions. Evidence from clinical experience also sets the stage for future research based on the more powerful and reliable tools of observational studies and randomized clinical trials.

To understand research findings or reports in the media, you must also be familiar with some basic ideas in medical research.

Every study must contend with variability in how participants respond to a treatment. Often people respond very differently indeed — a drug that is curative with few side effects for one person may do nothing but cause headaches or nausea in another. The best way to contend with variation is to observe large groups of people — in this way, extremes of response can be more easily spotted and a determination of an average or typical response can be made. (The number of study subjects in a study is called the sample size and is usually indicated with the letter N. Hence, $N =$ 345 means the study consists of 345 subjects.) In general, the smaller the sample, the less reliable the information from the study; however, deciding if a sample size is adequate is tricky and depends critically on the type of response expected in the study. These days researchers usually perform calculations ahead of time to determine a sample size large enough to allow them to detect a difference between the two groups.

Savvy health-care consumers also need to recognize that two items may seem to be linked yet do not have any actual cause-effect relationship. For example, the rate of smoking among depressed teenagers is higher than the rate among nondepressed teenagers.[1] Does this mean that smoking causes depression? Almost certainly not. This is an example of the old saying "Association does not equal causation." Smoking and depression are associated, but one does not cause the other.

Sometimes it can be very difficult to determine if a causal relationship exists between two phenomena. For example, controversy continues over the relationship between menopause and mood disorders. Early studies showed a link, and it seemed natural to think that the cause was low levels of estrogen — a "fact" used to help sell hormone replacement therapy. Later studies, however, questioned this "cause," pointing instead to evidence that the real culprits are a sudden change in hormone levels, not low levels per se, as well as the sleep disturbances caused by hot flashes. The jury is still out on this question — which only proves the difficulty in teasing apart association and causation.

Another important aspect of medical research is the difference between a result that is statistically significant and one that has practical significance to patients. A result is said to be statistically significant if it is highly unlikely to have been produced by the random variation inherent in all measurements. Using some basic statistical techniques, researchers can estimate the probability that a given result would occur by chance alone — a number called the p-value. P-values are always given as decimal equivalents to percentages. For example, if a given result would be expected to occur by chance 50 percent of the time (a very high p-value), the result would be reported as being "significant at $p = 0.5$." Clearly, such a result would not be very persuasive evidence, since it could as easily have resulted from random variation as from the actual treatment being explored.

Traditionally, medical researchers consider results that would only occur by chance one time out of twenty or, even better, one time out of one hundred, to be "statistically significant." Results with p-values lower than 0.05 (one out of twenty) or 0.01 (one out of a hundred), in other words, indicate strong evidence that a result was due to the treatment, not chance.

Just because a result is statistically significant, however, doesn't mean it has practical benefit. It's appropriate to ask a doctor whether he or she thinks that the results from a given study are clinically relevant or not.

When evaluating any health claim, whether in the course of a conversation or reading a media story or an article in a peer-reviewed journal, keep in mind the following questions:

- Were the results definitely published in a peer-reviewed journal?
- How many people were studied?
- If the study was a clinical trial, were patients randomized? If not, why not?
- Were study participants and researchers "blinded" during the study?
- Were people included or excluded from the study for particular reasons, and how many subjects, if any, dropped out during the course of the study?
- Who supported the study financially? (High-quality medical journals require that funders, which are often drug companies, disclose this fact and, in addition, that the study authors disclose any financial ties they might have to the funding agency. If a drug company sponsors an article that reports favorably on the company's drug, the results should be regarded with heightened scrutiny for potential bias or selective presentation of information.)

Media reports that cite the source of their information and specific details of the study (such as the sample size, funding source, and study methods) are more reliable than short reports of "results" from "clinical studies" about some aspect of medical research. Embracing a reasonable skepticism about findings reported in the media makes sense and can empower you in discussions with health-care providers.[2]

Appendix III

Medications That Can
Cause or Exacerbate
Anxiety and Depression

The range of prescribed medications today is vast, and inevitably, some have therapeutic properties or side effects that can either cause or exacerbate anxiety or depression. Commonly used substances such as alcohol, nicotine, and caffeine can have similar effects. Knowing about these potential effects can help one avoid anxiety and depression in the first place or recognize that troubling symptoms may be caused by a medication or drug rather than an underlying disorder.

The medicines listed in the table below do not cause or exacerbate anxiety for most people who take them, but they have the potential to do so in some individuals. Always consult a physician before making any changes in medications.

Medications with Possible Anxiety-Related Side Effects

DRUG	USED TO TREAT
Amphetamines, such as Dexadrine and Adderall	Child or adult attention deficit/hyperactivity disorder; relief of drowsiness or somnolence
Benztropine mesylate, such as Bensylate and Cogentin	Parkinson disease
Caffeine, such as NoDoz and Vivarin	Relief of drowsiness
Carbidopa, such as Sinemet and Lodosyn	Parkinson disease
Diphenhydramine hydrochloride, such as Allerdryl, Benadryl, Fenylhist, Nordryl, Nytol, and Sominex	Allergic responses, insomnia, coughs, motion sickness
Ephedrine, such as Ectasule, Efedron, Ephedsol, and Vatronol	Allergy-related congestion, asthma, relief of drowsiness
Epinephrine, such as Epifrin, Epinal, Eppy/N, and Glaucon	Asthma, allergic reactions, cardiac rhythm disturbances
Interferon, such as Avonex, Alferon N, Intron-A, Roferon-A, and Infergen	Antiviral agent and cancer chemotherapy

Medications with Possible Anxiety-Related Side Effects (*cont.*)

DRUG	USED TO TREAT
Levodopa (L-Dopa), such as Dopar and Larodopa	Parkinson disease
Parlodel (bromocriptine)	Suppression of lactation and Parkinson disease
Prednisone, such as Cortan, Deltasone, Liquid Pred, Meticorten, Orasone, Panasol-S, Prednicen-M, Prednisone Intensol	Swelling, rash, itching, allergic responses
Pseudoephedrine hydrochloride, such as Cenafed, Eltor, Halofed, Novafed, PediCare, Robidrine, Sudafed, and Sudrin	Decongestant
Symmetrel (amantadine)	Parkinson disease
Tricyclic antidepressants, such as Anafranil, Elavil, Tofranil, Pamelor, and Sinequan	Antidepressants

Depression is a relatively uncommon side effect of the drugs listed in the following table, but depressive responses occur often enough that both patients and physicians should be aware of the potential. Depressive symptoms should always be discussed with a doctor, and one should never discontinue or change the dose of a medication without prior approval. Note also that this list is not exhaustive but covers only the most widely used medications or medication categories with known potential to induce depressive symptoms.

Medications with Possible Depressive Side Effects

MEDICATION	USED TO TREAT
Accutane (isotretinoin)	Severe acne
Aldomet (methyldopa)	High blood pressure
Amipaque (metrizamide)	A medical dye used in certain radiology tests
Anticonvulsants, such as Celontin and Zanontin	Epileptic seizures
Barbiturates, such as phenobarbitol and secobarbitol	Insomnia, anxiety, muscle spasms
Benzodiazepines, such as Ativan, Dalmane, Halcion, Klonopin, Librium, Restoril, Valium, and Xanax	Insomnia, anxiety, muscle spasms
Beta-adrenergic blockers (beta-blockers), such as acebutolol, atenolol, bisoprolol, metoprolol, nadolol, propanolol, and timolol	Heart disease and migraine headache

Medications with Possible Depressive Side Effects (*cont.*)

MEDICATION	USED TO TREAT
Calcium-channel blockers, such as diltiazem, nifedipine, and verapamil	Heart disease
Corticosteroids, such as Azmacort, Clobetasol, Flonase, Flovent, Hydrocortisone, Nasocort, Nasonex, Methylprednisolone, Prednisone, and Triamcinolone	Swelling, rashes, allergies, and immune system disorders
Dapsone	Pneumonia and certain skin problems
Digoxin (digitalis)	Heart disease
Elspar (asparaginase)	Cancer
Estrogens, such as Premarin and Prempro	Menopause and prevention of osteoporosis
Flagyl (metronidazole)	Bacterial infections
Fluoroquinolone antibiotics, such as Levaquin	Respiratory tract infections
Histamine H_2-receptor antagonists, such as Axid, Mylanta, Pepcid, Tagamet, and Zantac	Ulcers, heartburn, and acid indigestion
Lariam (mefloquine)	Malaria
Lioresal (baclofen)	Muscle spasms
Narcotics, such as Codeine, Demerol, Darvocet, Morphine, and Percodan	Pain relief and cough suppression
Norpace (disopyramide)	Abnormal heart rhythm
Parlodel (bromocriptine)	Parkinson disease
Progestins such as Depo-Provera Norplant, Prempro, Premphase, Provera	Birth control, infertility, PMS
Reglan (metoclopramide)	Nausea and vomiting
Roferon-A (alfa interferon)	Certain cancers and chronic, active hepatitis B
Seromycin (cycloserine)	Tuberculosis
Statins (HMG-CoA reductase inhibitors), such as Lescol, Lipitor, Mevacor, Pravachol, and Zocor	High cholesterol treatment
Sulfonamides	Infections
Zovirax (acyclovir)	Shingles and herpes treatment

APPENDIX IV

FINDING HELP

Many types of people and organizations can provide accurate, reliable information about anxiety and depression and suggest appropriate doctors and psychotherapists:

- Talk to close family members and friends for their recommendations, especially if they have had a good experience with psychotherapy.
- Contact the psychiatry department of a nearby medical school or the psychology department of a local university.
- Contact a local hospital and ask about mental health clinics or staff psychiatrists.
- Ask a primary-care physician for a referral. Tell the doctor what's important to you in choosing a therapist so he or she can make appropriate suggestions.
- Inquire at a church, synagogue, or other faith-based organization.
- Look in the telephone book for a local mental health association or a state or provincial department of mental health. Check these sources for possible referrals.
- Investigate the websites of the organizations listed in this appendix.

For information specifically about anxiety and depression in children and teens, along with many resources for finding doctors and therapists in a particular region, contact the American Academy of Child and Adolescent Psychiatry.

Address: 3615 Wisconsin Avenue, NW, Washington, DC 20016-3007
Phone: 202-966-7300
Web address: http://www.aacap.org

To find a behavioral therapist, contact the Association for Advancement of Behavior Therapy.

Address: 305 Seventh Avenue, 16th Floor, New York, NY 10001-6008
Phone: 212-647-1890
Web address: www.aabt.org/CLINICAL/CLINICAL.HTM

To find a cognitive therapist, contact the Academy of Cognitive Therapy.

Address: 1 Belmont Avenue, Suite 700, Bala Cynwyd, PA 19004
Phone: 610-664-1273
Web address: www.academyofct.org/Info/CertifiedMembers.asp (This site also has a state-by-state list of low-cost cognitive therapists.)

Although hundreds of groups and organizations focus on anxiety, depression, or both, few meet the highest standards for evidence-based, peer-reviewed, and regularly updated information. The following organizations, listed alphabetically, meet these standards.

Association for the Advancement of Behavior Therapy

Address: 305 Seventh Avenue, 16th Floor, New York, NY 10001-6008
Phone: 212-647-1890
Web address: www.aabt.org

American Foundation for Suicide Prevention

Address: 120 Wall Street, 22nd Floor, New York, NY 10005
Phone: 888-333-2377
Web address: www.afsp.org

American Psychiatric Association

Address: 1000 Wilson Boulevard, Suite 1825, Arlington, VA 22209-3901
Phone: 703-907-7300
Web address: www.psych.org

American Psychological Association

Address: 750 First Street, NE, Washington, DC 20002-4242
Phone: 800-374-2721 or 202-336-5510
Web address: www.apa.org

Anxiety Disorders Association of America

Address: 8730 Georgia Avenue, Suite 600, Silver Spring, MD 20910
Phone: 240-485-1001
Web address: www.adaa.org

Center for Mental Health Services

Web address: www.mentalhealth.org

Child and Adolescent Bipolar Association

Address: 1187 Wilmette Avenue, PMB #331, Wilmette, IL 60091
Phone: 847-256-8525
Web address: www.bpkids.org

Depression After Delivery, Inc.

Address: 91 East Somerset Street, Raritan, NJ 08869
Phone: 800-944-4773
Web address: www.depressionafterdelivery.com

Depression and Bipolar Support Alliance

Address: 730 N. Franklin Street, Suite 501, Chicago, IL 60610-7204
Phone: 800-826-3632
Web address: www.dbsalliance.org

Freedom from Fear

Address: 308 Seaview Avenue, Staten Island, NY 10305
Phone: 718-351-1717
Web address: www.freedomfromfear.com

The Jed Foundation
(A nonprofit organization dedicated to reducing college-age suicide)

Address: 583 Broadway, Suite 8B, New York, NY 10012
Phone: 212-343-0016
Web address: www.jedfoundation.org

National Alliance for the Mentally Ill

Address: Colonial Place Three, 2107 Wilson Boulevard, Suite 300,
Arlington, VA 22201
Phone: 800-950-6264 or 703-524-7600
Web address: www.nami.org

National Alliance for Research on Schizophrenia and Depression

Address: 60 Cutter Mill Road, Suite 404. Great Neck, New York 11021
Phone: 516-829-0091
Web address: www.nasrad.org

NATIONAL CENTER FOR POSTTRAUMATIC STRESS DISORDER

Address: U.S. Department of Veterans Affairs, 116D VA Medical and
Regional Office Center, 215 N. Main Street, White River Junction, VT
05009
Phone: 802-296-6300
Web address: www.ncptsd.org

NATIONAL INSTITUTE OF MENTAL HEALTH

Address: 6001 Executive Boulevard, Room 8184, MSC 9663, Bethesda,
MD 20892-9663
Phone: 301-443-4513
General Web address: www.nimh.nih.gov
For information on anxiety: www.nimh.nih.gov/anxiety/
anxietymenu.cfm
For information on depression: www.nimh.nih.gov/publicat/
depressionmenu.cfm

National Mental Health Association

Address: 2001 N. Beauregard Street, 12th Floor, Alexandria, VA 22311
Phone: 800-969-6642 or 703-684-7722
Web address: www.nmha.org

Obsessive-Compulsive Foundation

Address: 337 Notch Hill Road, North Branford, CT 06471
Phone: 203-315-2190
Web address: www.ocfoundation.org

Parents Without Partners

Address: 1650 South Dixie Highway, Suite 510, Boca Raton, FL 33432
Phone: 561-391-8833
Web address: http://www.parentswithoutpartners.org

Heinz C. Prechter Fund for Manic Depression

Address: One Heritage Place, Suite 400, Southgate, MI 48195
Phone 734-246-0056
Web address: www.hcpfmd.org

Stanley Medical Research Institute

Address: 5430 Grosvenor Lane, Suite 200, Bethesda, Maryland 20814
Phone: 301-571-0760
Web address: www. stanleyresearch.org

Teen Central

Phone: 800-334-4KID
Web address: http://teencentral.net

APPENDIX V

WHO DOES WHAT?

The range of people who treat psychological conditions is wide and can be confusing. As yet no national standards or national licenses exist in the field of mental health. Each state decides whether a license is needed to call oneself a "therapist," what specific types of mental health workers need to be licensed and what standards they must uphold to keep their licenses, and the procedures and precipitating actions involved in revoking a license. Wide variation therefore exists in the skills and experience of mental health workers. Although psychiatrists, in general, have a more standardized training than other mental health workers, we recommend limiting yourself to psychiatrists who are also certified by the American Board of Psychiatry and Neurology. See Appendix IV for information on finding mental health workers.

These are the kinds of mental health professionals one might contact for help with anxiety or depression, listed here roughly in order of the amount of specialized training required to practice.

- PSYCHIATRISTS are medical doctors and have completed at least four years of additional training in psychiatric disorders following medical school. They are the only mental health workers who can prescribe medications. The American Board of Psychiatry and Neurology certifies psychiatrists based on written and oral examinations.
- PSYCHOLOGISTS have specialized training in psychological disorders and treatment, and have doctoral degrees (a Ph.D., Psy.D., or Ed.D.). They frequently treat a range of conditions with any of various forms of psychotherapy and will refer a person to a psychiatrist if medications seem warranted.
- PSYCHOANALYSTS are usually psychiatrists or psychologists who specialize in the psychotherapy called psychoanalysis, pioneered by Sigmund Freud. Psychoanalysis focuses on identifying unconscious

feelings, needs, conflicts, or barriers to healthy mental function. Psychoanalytic institutes provide certification after completion of psychoanalytic training.

- **CLINICAL OR PSYCHIATRIC SOCIAL WORKERS** have at least a master's degree in social work and specialized training in psychology and psychotherapy. They often deal with family or interpersonal problems.

- **COUNSELORS** assist people with personal, family, educational, mental health, financial, and career decisions or problems. They may not have formal or accredited training in psychotherapy. Their duties depend on the individuals they serve and on the settings in which they work.

- **THERAPISTS** fill a variety of roles. The term *therapist* is so generic and widely used that a single definition is not possible. Therapists may or may not have formal training or certification by a professional organization or be qualified to treat psychological disorders.

- **PASTORAL COUNSELORS** are religious leaders whose counseling practice integrates religious traditions with insights from the behavioral sciences. Some pastoral counselors complete a course of training and observation and are certified by the American Association of Pastoral Counselors.

- **LAY COUNSELORS** are member volunteers of a religious organization who care for and support others. They often have attended training programs or workshops that equip them to discern when an individual needs the attention of a psychiatrist or other doctor.

Notes

Introduction: Empowering People with Anxiety and Depression

1. C.J.L. Murray and A. D. Lopez, eds., *Summary: The Global Burden of Disease: A Comprehensive Assessment of Mortality and Disability from Diseases, Injuries, and Risk Factors in 1990 and Projected to 2020* (Cambridge, Mass.: Harvard University Press, 1996). Published by the Harvard School of Public Health on behalf of the World Health Organization and the World Bank.
2. W. F. Steward, J. A. Ricci, E. Chee, et al., "Cost of Lost Productive Work Time Among U.S. Workers with Depression," *Journal of the American Medical Association (JAMA)* 289 (2003): 3135–43.
3. M. Olfson, S. C. Marcus, and B. Druss, "National Trends in the Outpatient Treatment of Depression," *JAMA* 287 (2002): 203–9.
4. National Institute of Mental Health, *The Numbers Count: Mental Disorders in America* (Bethesda, Md.: NIMH, January 2001), NIMH Publication No. 01-4584.
5. Dennis S. Charney has received research grants in the past from the following companies: Forest Laboratories Aventis and GlaxoSmithKline. He has in the past served as a paid consultant to the following companies: Abbott Laboratories, Bristol-Myers Squibb, Forest Laboratories, Eli Lilly, GlaxoSmithKline, Janssen Pharmaceutica, Merck, Novartis, Organon, Somerset, and Wyeth-Ayerst. He currently serves as a consultant to AstraZeneca, Otsuka, and Cyberonics.

Charles B. Nemeroff has received research grants from the following companies: Abbott Laboratories, AFSP, AstraZeneca, Bristol-Myers Squibb, Eli Lilly, Forest Laboratories, GlaxoSmithKline, Janssen Pharmaceutica, Merck, NARSAD, NIMH, Pfizer, Stanley Foundation/NAMI, and Wyeth-Ayerst. He has served as a paid consultant to the following companies: Abbott Laboratories, Acadia Pharmaceuticals, AstraZeneca, Bristol-Myers Squibb, Corcept, Cypress Biosciences, Cyberonics, Eli Lilly, Forest Laboratories, GlaxoSmithKline, Janssen Pharmaceutica, Merck, Neurocrine Biosciences, Novartis,

Organon, Otsuka, Sanofi, Scirex, Somerset, and Wyeth-Ayerst. He is a member of the speakers bureau for the following companies: Abbott Laboratories, AstraZeneca, Bristol-Myers Squibb, Eli Lilly, Forest Laboratories, GlaxoSmithKline, Janssen Pharmaceutica, Organon, Otsuka, Pfizer, and Wyeth-Ayerst. He is a stockholder in the following companies: Corcept and Neurocrine Biosciences. He has the following patents related to the treatment of anxiety or depression: method and devices for transdermal delivery of lithium (US 6,375,990 B1); method to estimate serotonin and norepinephrine transporter occupancy after drug treatment using patient or animal serum (provisional filing April 2001).

6. R. C. Kessler, P. Berglund, O. Demler, et al., "The Epidemiology of Major Depressive Disorder," *JAMA* 289, 23 (2003): 3095–3105.

7. J. Rapoport, *The Boy Who Couldn't Stop Washing: The Experience and Treatment of Obsessive-Compulsive Disorder* (New York: HarperCollins, 1990.)

1. THIEVES OF HAPPINESS

1. J. Angst, "Depression and Anxiety: Implications for Nosology, Course, and Treatment," *Journal of Clinical Psychiatry* 58 (Suppl. 8) (1997): 3–5.

2. This story is based on information presented in the article "Experimental Study of a Case of Insensitivity to Pain," by G. A. McMurray, *Archives of Neurology and Psychiatry* 64 (1950): 650–67.

3. M. McGuire and A. Troisi, *Darwinian Psychiatry* (New York: Oxford University Press, 1998).

4. W. C. Drevets, K. M. Gadde, K. Ranga, and K. Krishman, "Neuroimaging Studies of Mood Disorders," in *Neurobiology of Mental Illness*, 2nd edition, ed. D. S. Charney and E. J. Nestler (New York: Oxford University Press, 2004); H. Mayberg, "Reciprocal Limbic-Cortical Function and Negative Mood: Converging PET Findings in Depression and Normal Sadness," *American Journal of Psychiatry* 156 (1999): 675–82.

5. D. S. Charney, D. H. Barlow, K. Botteron, et al., "Neuroscience Research Agenda to Guide Development of a Pathophysiologically Based Classification System," in *A Research Agenda for DSM-V*, ed. D. J. Kupfer, M. B. First, D. A. Regier, and M. F. Schachter (Washington, D.C.: American Psychiatric Press, 2002).

2. BUILDING EMOTIONAL RESILIENCE

1. A. S. Masten, "Ordinary Magic: Resilience Processes in Development," *American Psychologist* 56 (2001): 227–38.

2. D. S. Charney, "Psychobiological Mechanisms of Resilience and Vulnerabil-

ity: Implications for the Successful Adaptation to Extreme Stress." *American Journal of Psychiatry* 161 (2) (2004) Feb. 1.

3. T. C. Seeman, B. S. McEwen, J. W. Rowe, and B. H. Singer, "Allostatic Load as a Marker of Cumulative Biological Risk: MacArthur Studies of Successful Aging," *Proceedings of the National Academy of Science, USA* 98 (2001): 4470–75.

4. C. W. Cotman and N. C. Berchtold, "Exercise: A Behavioral Intervention to Enhance Brain Health and Plasticity," *Trends in Neuroscience* 25, 6 (2002): 295–301.

5. R. Adolphs, "Cognitive Neuroscience of Human Social Behavior," *Nature Reviews: Neuroscience* 4 (2003): 165–78.

6. J. Bowlby, *A Secure Base: Parent-Child Attachment and Healthy Human Development* (New York: Basic Books, 1988).

7. M. Rutter, "The Interplay of Nature, Nurture, and Developmental Influences," *Archives of General Psychiatry* 59 (2002): 996–1000.

8. E. S. Epel, B. S. McEwen, and J. R. Ickovics, "Embodying Psychological Thriving: Physical Thriving in Response to Stress," *Journal of Social Issues* 54, 2 (1998): 301–22.

9. R. Janoff-Bulman and C. M. Frantz, "The Loss of Illusions: The Potent Legacy of Trauma," *Journal of Personal and Interpersonal Loss* 1 (1996): 133–50.

10. T. Shantall, *Life's Meaning in the Face of Suffering: Testimonies of Holocaust Survivors* (Jerusalem: Manges Press, Hebrew University, 2002).

11. C. L. Katz and R. Nathaniel, "Disasters, Psychiatry, and Psychodynamics," *Journal of the American Academy of Psychoanalysis* 30, 4 (2002): 519–29.

12. Masten, "Ordinary Magic."

13. D. Lykken, *Happiness: What Studies on Twins Show Us About Nature, Nurture, and the Happiness Set Point* (New York: Golden Books, 1999).

14. R. G. Tedeschi, C. L. Park, and L. G. Calhoun, eds., *Posttraumatic Growth: Positive Changes in the Aftermath of Crisis* (Mahwah, N.J.: Erlbaum, 1998).

15. Ibid.

16. G. E. Richardson, "The Metatheory of Resilience and Resiliency," *Journal of Clinical Psychology* 58, 3 (2002): 307–21.

3. Mood and Physical Health

1. V. Benson and M. A. Marano, "Current Estimates from the National Health Interview Survey, 1995, National Center for Health Statistics," *Vital Health Statistics* 10, 199 (1998).

2. F. Lesperance, N. Frasure-Smith, and M. Taljic, "Major Depression Before and After Myocardial Infarction: Its Nature and Consequences," *Psychosomatic Medicine* 58 (1996): 99–110.

3. K. R. Krishnan, M. Delong, H. Kraemer, et al., "Comorbidity of Depression

with Other Medical Diseases in the Elderly," *Biological Psychiatry* 52, 6 (2002): 559–88.

4. L. D. Kubzansky, I. Kawachi, S. T. Weiss, and D. Sparrow, "Anxiety and Coronary Heart Disease: A Synthesis of Epidemiological, Psychological, and Experimental Evidence," *Annals of Behavioral Medicine* 20, 2 (Spring 1998): 47–58.

5. R. M. Carney and K. E. Freedland, "Depression, Mortality, and Medical Morbidity in Patients with Coronary Heart Disease," *Biological Psychiatry* 54, 3 (2003): 241–47.

6. S. P. Roose, "Treatment of Depression in Patients with Heart Disease," *Biological Psychiatry* 54, 3 (2003): 262–68.

7. Writing committee for the ENRICHD investigators, "Effects of Treating Depression and Low Perceived Social Support on Clinical Events After Myocardial Infarction," *JAMA* 289 (2003): 3106–16.

8. Krishnan et al., "Comorbidity of Depression."

9. D. L. Evans and D. S. Charney, "Mood Disorders and Medical Illness: A Major Public Health Problem," *Biological Psychiatry* 54, 3 (2003): 177–80.

10. R. G. Robinson, "Poststroke Depression: Prevalence, Diagnosis, Treatment, and Disease Progression," *Biological Psychiatry* 54, 3 (2003): 376–87.

11. *Diabetes Statistics* (Bethesda, Md.: National Institute of Diabetes and Digestive and Kidney Diseases, March 1999), NIH Pub. No. 99-3892.

12. R. J. Anderson, P. J. Lustman, R. E. Clouse, et al., "Prevalence of Depression in Adults with Diabetes: A Systematic Review," *Diabetes* 49 (Suppl. 1) (2000): A64.

13. G. Cizza, P. Ravn, G. P. Chrousos, et al., "Depression: A Major, Unrecognized Risk Factor for Osteoporosis?" *Trends in Endocrinology and Metabolism* 12, 5 (2001): 198–203.

14. National Osteoporosis Foundation "Disease Facts" page. Available at www.nof.org/osteoporosis/stats.htm. Accessed Jan. 29, 2003.

15. M. A. Whooley, K. E. Kip, J. A. Cauley, et al., "Depression, Falls, and Risk of Fracture in Older Women: Study of Osteoporotic Fractures Research Group," *Archives of Internal Medicine* 159, 5 (1999): 484–90.

16. J. Leserman, E. D. Jackson, J. M. Petitto, et al., "Progression to AIDS: The Effects of Stress, Depressive Symptoms, and Social Support," *Psychosomatic Medicine* 61, 3 (1999): 397–406.

17. M. M. Ohayon and A. F. Schatzberg, "Using Chronic Pain to Predict Depressive Morbidity in the General Population," *Archives of General Psychiatry* 60, 1 (2003): 39–47.

18. D. L. Musselman, D. H. Lawson, J. F. Gumnick, et al., "Paroxetine for the Prevention of Depression Induced by High-Dose Interferon Alfa," *New England Journal of Medicine* 344, 13 (Mar. 29, 2001): 961–66.

19. C. L. Raison and A. H. Miller, "Depression in Cancer: New Developments Regarding Diagnosis and Treatment," *Biological Psychiatry* 54, 3 (2003): 283–94.

20. D. Spiegel, "Cancer and Depression," *British Medical Journal* 168 (1996): 109–16.
21. D. L. Evans, J. P. Staab, J. M. Petitto, et al., "Depression in the Medical Setting: Biopsychological Interactions and Treatment Considerations," *Journal of Clinical Psychiatry* 60 (1999): 40–45.
22. B. W. Penninx, J. M. Guralnik, M. Pahor, et al., "Chronically Depressed Mood and Cancer Risk in Older Persons," *Journal of the National Cancer Institute* 90 (1998): 1888–93; K. Hjerl, E. W. Andersen, N. Keiding, et al., "Depression as a Prognostic Factor for Breast Cancer Mortality," *Psychosomatics* 44, 1 (Jan.–Feb. 2003): 24–30.
23. D. Spiegel and J. Giese-Davis, "Depression and Cancer: Mechanisms and Disease Progression," *Biological Psychiatry* 54, 3 (2003): 269–82.
24. B. S. McEwen, "Mood Disorders and Allostatic Load," *Biological Psychiatry* 54, 3 (2003): 200–207.

4. THE WORLD OF ANXIETY DISORDERS

1. W. E. Narrow, D. S. Rae, and D. A. Regier, "NIMH Epidemiology Note: Prevalence of Anxiety Disorders," one-year prevalence best estimates calculated from ECA and NCS data. Population estimates based on U.S. Census estimated residential population ages 18 to 54 on July 1, 1998.
2. R. R. Crowe, "Molecular Genetics of Anxiety Disorders," in *Neurobiology of Mental Illness*, 2nd edition, ed. D. S. Charney and E. J. Nestler (New York: Oxford University Press, 2004), 451–62.
3. Ibid.
4. J. M. Hettema, P. Annas, M. C. Neale, et al., "A Twin Study of the Genetics of Fear Conditioning," *Archives of General Psychiatry* 60, 7 (2003): 702–8.
5. S. P. Hamilton, A. J. Fyer, M. Durner, et al., "Further Genetic Evidence for a Panic Disorder Syndrome Mapping to Chromosome 13q," *Proceedings of the National Academy of Science* 100, 5 (2003): 2550–55.
6. K. Alsene, J. Deckert, P. Sand, and H. de Wit, "Association Between A2a Receptor Gene Polymorphisms and Caffeine-Induced Anxiety," *Neuropsychopharmacology* 28, 9 (2003): 1694–1702.
7. J. M. Neiderhiser, D. Reiss, R. Plomin, et al., "Relationships Between Parenting and Adolescent Adjustment over Time: Genetic and Environmental Contributions," *Developmental Psychology* 35, 3 (1999): 680–92.
8. M. J. Essex, M. H. Klein, E. Cho, et al., "Maternal Stress Beginning in Infancy May Sensitize Children to Later Stress Exposure: Effects on Cortisol and Behavior," *Biological Psychiatry* 52 (2002): 776–84.
9. A. S. Masten, "Ordinary Magic: Resilience Processes in Development," *American Psychologist* 56 (2001): 227–38.
10. J. M. Gorman, S. Mathew, and J. Coplan, "Neurobiology of Early Life Stress:

Nonhuman Primate Models," *Seminars in Clinical Neuropsychiatry* 7, 2 (2002): 96–103.

11. Ricky Williams's story here is based on the following public accounts of his struggle with general anxiety disorder: GlaxoSmithKline press release, May 1, 2003; Thomas George, "Emerging from the Shadows," *New York Times,* July 24, 2002; statistics sheet provided by Cohn & Wolfe Company as part of national publicity tour by Williams and Terry Bradshaw; Alex Marvez, "The Man Behind the Mask," *Sports Illustrated for Kids,* Jan. 1, 2003; interview with Williams, www.paxil.com, accessed June 17, 2003.

12. Narrow et al., "NIMH Epidemiology Note."

13. D. A. Regier, D. S. Rae, W. E. Narrow, et al., "Prevalence of Anxiety Disorders and Their Comorbidity with Mood and Addictive Disorders," *British Journal of Psychiatry* (Suppl. 34) (1998): 24–28.

14. M. S. Marcin and C. B. Nemeroff, "The Neurobiology of Social Phobia: The Relevance of Fear and Anxiety," *Acta Psychiatrica Scandinavica* 417 (Suppl.) (2003): 51–64.

15. M. B. Stein, P. R. Goldin, J. Sareen, et al., "Increased Amygdala Activation to Angry and Contemptuous Faces in Generalized Social Phobia," *Archives of General Psychiatry* 59, 11 (2002): 1027–34.

16. N. Brunello, J. R. Davidson, M. Deahl, R. C. Kessler, et al., "Posttraumatic Stress Disorder: Diagnosis and Epidemiology, Comorbidity and Social Consequences, Biology and Treatment," *Neuropsychobiology* 43, 3 (2001): 150–62.

17. J. D. Bremner, P. Randall, E. Vermetten, et al., "Magnetic Resonance Imaging–Based Measurement of Hippocampal Volume in Posttraumatic Stress Disorder Related to Childhood Physical and Sexual Abuse — A Preliminary Report," *Biological Psychiatry* 41 (1997): 23–32.

18. J. Przybyslawski, P. Roullet, and S. J. Sara, "Attenuation of Emotional and Non-emotional Memories After Their Re-activation: Role of Beta Adrenergic Receptors," *Neuroscience* 19 (1999): 6623–28.

19. S. L. Rauch, L. M. Shin, E. Segal, et al., "Selectively Reduced Regional Cortical Volumes in Post-Traumatic Stress Disorder," *Neuroreport* 14, 7 (2003): 913–16.

20. Narrow et al., "NIMH Epidemiology Note."

21. H.-U. Wittchen, S. Zhao, R. C. Kessler, and W. W. Eaton, "DSM-III-R Generalized Anxiety Disorder in the National Comorbidity Survey," *Archives of General Psychiatry* 51 (1994): 355–64.

22. D. H. Barlow, B. F. Chorpita, and J. Turovsky, "Fear, Panic, Anxiety, and Disorders of Emotion," in *Perspectives on Anxiety, Panic, and Fear,* ed. D. A. Hope (Lincoln: Nebraska University Press, 1996), 251–328.

23. American Psychiatric Association, "Practice Guidelines for the Treatment of Patients with Panic Disorder," *American Journal of Psychiatry* 155 (Suppl. 12) (1998): 1–34.

24. D. S. Charney and J. D. Bremner, "The Neurobiology of Anxiety Disorders,"

in *Neurobiology of Mental Illness*, 2nd edition, ed. D. S. Charney and E. J. Nestler (New York: Oxford University Press, 2004): 605–27.

25. M. B. Stein and W. U. Thomas, "Biology of Anxiety Disorders," in *Textbook of Psychopharmacology*, ed. A. F. Schatzberg and C. B. Nemeroff (Washington, D.C.: American Psychiatric Press, 1998), 609–28.

26. J. M. Woo, K. S. Yoon, and B. H. Yu, "Catechol O-methyltransferase Genetic Polymorphism in Panic Disorder," *American Journal of Psychiatry* 159, 10 (2002): 1785–87.

5. FINDING OPTIMAL RELIEF FROM ANXIETY DISORDERS

1. C. B. Taylor, "Treatment of Anxiety Disorders," in *Textbook of Psychopharmacology*, ed. A. F. Schatzberg and C. B. Nemeroff (Washington, D.C.: American Psychiatric Press, 1998).

2. A. W. Goddard et al., "Early Co-administration of Clonazepam with Sertraline for Panic Disorder," *Archives of General Psychiatry* 58 (2001): 681–86.

3. The following SSRIs present generally lower risks for metabolic interference than other SSRIs do: Zoloft (sertraline), Paxil (paroxetine), and Celexa (citalopram). The benzodiazepines Xanax (alprazolam), Valium (diazepam), Ativan (lorazepam), Serax (oxazepam), and Restoril (temazepam) are less likely to have metabolic interactions with SSRIs than are other benzodiazepines.

4. I. Marks, K. Lovell, H. Noshirvani, et al., "Treatment of Posttraumatic Stress Disorder by Exposure and/or Cognitive Restructuring: A Controlled Study," *Archives of General Psychiatry* 55, 4 (1998): 317–25.

5. E. B. Foa, J.R.T. Davidson, and A. Frances, eds., "The Expert Consensus Guideline Series: Treatment of Posttraumatic Stress Disorder," *Journal of Clinical Psychiatry* 60 (Suppl. 16) (1999).

6. E. R. Peskind, L. T. Bonner, D. J. Hoff, and M. A. Raskind, "Prazosin Reduces Trauma-Related Nightmares in Older Men with Chronic Posttraumatic Stress Disorder," *Journal of Geriatric Psychiatry and Neurology* 16, 3 (2003): 165–71.

7. C. R. Marmar, T. C. Neylan, and F. B. Schoenfeld, "New Directions in the Pharmacotherapy of Posttraumatic Stress Disorder," *Psychiatric Quarterly* 73, 4 (2002): 259–70.

8. J. LeDoux, *The Emotional Brain* (New York: Simon & Schuster, 1996).

9. F. A. Goodyear-Smith, T. M. Laidlaw, and R. G. Large, "Memory Recovery and Repression: What Is the Evidence?" *Health Care Analysis* 5, 2 (1997): 99–111.

10. American Psychological Association position paper on recovered memories, at www.apa.org/pubinfo/mem.html. Accessed Feb. 14, 2003.

11. D. H. Barlow, J. M. Gorman, M. K. Shear, and S. W. Woods, "Cognitive-Be-

havioral Therapy, Imipramine, or Their Combination for Panic Disorder: A Randomized Controlled Trial," *JAMA* 283, 19 (2000): 2529–36.

6. The World of Depression

1. W. Styron, *Darkness Visible* (New York: Vintage, 1990), 16–17.
2. L. P. Riso, P. L. du Toit, J. A. Blandino, et al., "Cognitive Aspects of Chronic Depression," *Journal of Abnormal Psychology* 112, 1 (2003): 72–80.
3. R. Elliott, B. J. Sahakian, A. P. McKay, et al., "Neuropsychological Impairments in Unipolar Depression: The Influence of Perceived Failure on Subsequent Performance," *Psychological Medicine* 26, 5 (1996): 975–89.
4. C. M. Mazure and P. K. Maciejewski, "A Model of Risk for Major Depression: Effects of Life Stress and Cognitive Style Vary by Age," *Depression and Anxiety* 17, 1 (2003): 26–33.
5. L. E. Rosenberg, "Brainsick: A Physician's Journey to the Brink," *Cerebrum* 4, 4 (2002): 43–60.
6. American Psychiatric Association, *Diagnostic and Statistical Manual of Mental Disorders,* 4th ed. (Washington, D.C.: American Psychiatric Association Press, 1994).
7. A. J. Rothschild, "Challenges in the Treatment of Depression with Psychotic Features," *Biological Psychiatry* 53 (2003): 680–90.
8. American Psychiatric Association, "Practice Guideline for the Treatment of Major Depressive Disorder (Revision)," *American Journal of Psychiatry* (Suppl. 157) (2000): Suppl. 4.
9. P. C. Whybrow, *A Mood Apart: Depression, Mania, and Other Afflictions of the Self* (New York: Basic Books, 1997).
10. J. Angst, A. Gamma, and R. Sellaro, "Toward Validation of Atypical Depression in the Community: Results of the Zurich Cohort Study," *Journal of Affective Disorders* 72, 2 (2002): 125–38.
11. M. A. Posternak and M. Zimmerman, "Symptoms of Atypical Depression," *Psychiatry Research* 104, 2 (2001): 175–81.
12. P. J. McGrath, J. W. Stewart, and M. N. Janal, "A Placebo-Controlled Study of Fluoxetine Versus Imipramine in the Acute Treatment of Atypical Depression," *American Journal of Psychiatry* 157, 3 (2000): 344–50.
13. K. S. Kendler, C. A. Prescott, J. Myers, and M. C. Neale, "The Structure of Genetic and Environmental Risk Factors for Common Psychiatric and Substance Use Disorders in Men and Women," *Archives of General Psychiatry* 60, 9 (2003): 929–37.
14. A. Caspi, K. Sugden, T. E. Moffitt, et al., "Influence of Life Stress on Depression: Moderation by a Polymorphism in the 5-HTT Gene," *Science* 301 (2003): 386–89.
15. G. S. Zubenko, H. B. Hughes III, J. S. Stiffler, et al., "Sequence Variations in

CREB1 Cosegregate with Depressive Disorders in Women," *Molecular Psychiatry* 8, 6 (2003): 611–18.

16. A. J. Van der Does, "Acute Tryptophan Depletion Induces Depressive Symptoms in Subgroups of Recovered Depressed Patients," *Psychological Medicine* 33, 6 (2003): 1133–34.

17. M. Nibuya, E. J. Nestler, and R. S. Duman, "Chronic Antidepressant Administration Increases the Expression of cAMP Response Element Binding Protein (CREB) in Rat Hippocampus," *Journal of Neuroscience* 16, 7 (1996): 2365–72.

18. L. Arborelius, J. M. Owens, P. M. Plotsky, and C. B. Nemeroff, "The Role of Corticotropin-Releasing Factor in Depression and Anxiety Disorders," *Journal of Endocrinology* 160 (1999): 1–12.

19. R. S. Duman, "The Neurochemistry of Mood Disorders: Preclinical Studies," in *Neurobiology of Mental Illness*, 2nd edition, ed. D. S. Charney and E. J. Nestler (New York: Oxford University Press, 2004).

20. E. Frank, B. Anderson, C. F. Reynolds, et al., "Life Events and the Research Diagnostic Criteria Endogenous Subtype: A Confirmation of the Distinction Using the Bedford College Methods," *Archives of General Psychiatry* 51 (1994): 519–24; R. E. Ingram, J. Miranda, and Z. V. Segal, *Cognitive Vulnerability to Depression* (New York: Guilford, 1998).

21. J. M. Neiderhiser, D. Reiss, R. Plomin, et al., "Relationships Between Parenting and Adolescent Adjustment Over Time: Genetic and Environmental Contributions," *Developmental Psychology* 35, 3 (1999): 680–92.

22. A. Solomon, *The Noonday Demon: An Atlas of Depression* (New York: Touchstone, 2002).

23. H. G. Prigerson, P. K. Maciejewski, and R. A. Rosenhoek, "Preliminary Explorations of the Harmful Interactive Effects of Widowhood on Health Service Use and Health Care Costs," *Gerontologist* 40, 3 (2000): 373–78.

7. Finding Optimal Relief from Both Major and Low-Level Depression

1. National Advisory Mental Health Council, "Health Care Reform for Americans with Severe Mental Illnesses," *American Journal of Psychiatry* 150, 10 (1993): 1447–65.

2. R. M. Berman, J. K. Belanoff, D. S. Charney, and A. F. Schatzberg, "Principles of the Pharmacotherapy of Depression," in *Neurobiology of Mental Illness*, in *Neurobiology of Mental Illness*, ed. D. S. Charney and E. J. Nestler (New York: Oxford University Press, 2004).

3. S. E. Hyman and M. V. Rudorfer, "Depressive and Bipolar Mood Disorders," in *Scientific American Medicine, Vol. 3*, ed. D. C. Dale and D. D. Federman (New York: Healtheon/WebMD, 2000), sec. 13, p. 1.

4. C. B. Nemeroff, C. M. Heim, M. E. Thase, et al., "Differential Responses to Psychotherapy Versus Pharmacotherapy in the Treatment of Patients with Chronic Forms of Major Depression and Childhood Trauma," *Proceedings of the National Academy of Sciences* 100 (2003): 14293–96.

5. C. B. Nemeroff and A. F. Schatzberg, "Pharmacological Treatments for Unipolar Depression," in *A Guide to Treatments That Work*, 3d ed., ed. P. E. Nathan and J. M. Gorman (Washington, D.C.: American Psychiatric Association Press, 2003).

6. J. R. Geddes, S. M. Carney, C. Davies, et al., "Relapse Prevention with Antidepressant Drug Treatment in Depressive Disorders: A Systematic Review," *Lancet* 361 (2003): 653–61.

7. M. G. Warshaw and M. B. Keller, "The Relationship Between Fluoxetine Use and Suicidal Behavior in 654 Subjects with Anxiety Disorders," *Journal of Clinical Psychiatry* 57, 4 (1996): 158–66; S. S. Jick, A. D. Dean, and H. Jick, "Antidepressants and Suicide," *British Medical Journal* 310, 6974 (Jan. 28, 1995): 215–18.

8. C. B. Nemeroff, A. F. Schatzberg, D. J. Goldstein, et al., "Duloxetine for the Treatment of Major Depressive Disorder," *Psychopharmacology Bulletin* 36, 4 (2002): 106–32.

9. Ibid.

10. Nemeroff and Schatzberg, "Pharmacological Treatments."

11. D. S. Charney, R. M. Berman, and H. L. Miller, "Treatment of Depression," in *Textbook of Psychopharmacology*, 2d ed., ed. A. F. Schatzberg and C. B. Nemeroff (Washington, D.C.: American Psychiatric Press, 1998).

12. C. DeBattista, H. B. Solvason, J. Poirier, E. Kendrick, and A. F. Schatzberg, "A Prospective Trial of Bupropion SR Augmentation of Partial and Non-Responders to Serotonergic Antidepressants," *Journal of Clinical Psychopharmacology* 23, 1 (2003): 27–30.

13. F.J.L. Ruwe, R. A. Smulders, H. J. Kleijn, et al., "Mirtazapine and Paroxetine: A Drug-Drug Interaction Study in Healthy Subjects," *Human Psychopharmacology* 16 (2001): 449–59.

14. R. C. Shelton, G. D. Tollefson, M. Tohen, et al., "A Novel Augmentation Strategy for Treating Resistant Major Depression," *American Journal of Psychiatry* 158 (2001): 131–34.

15. J. Angst, "Natural History and Epidemiology of Depression," in *Results of Community Studies in Prediction and Treatment of Recurrent Depression*, ed. J. Cobb and N. Goeting (Southampton, Eng.: Duphar Medical Relations, 1990).

16. E. Frank, D. J. Kupfer, J. M. Perel, et al., "Three-Year Outcomes for Maintenance Therapies in Recurrent Depression," *Archives of General Psychiatry* 47 (1990): 1093–99.

17. K. Linde et al., "Saint John's Wort for Depression — An Overview and Meta-Analysis of Randomized Clinical Trials," *British Medical Journal* 313 (1996): 253–58.

18. R. C. Shelton, M. B. Keller, A. J. Gelenberg, et al., "Effectiveness of Saint John's Wort in Major Depression," *JAMA* 285 (2001): 1978–86; Hypericum Depression Trial Study Group, "Effect of *Hypericum perforatum* (Saint John's Wort) in Major Depressive Disorder: A Randomized, Controlled Trial," *JAMA* 287 (2002): 1807–14.

19. J. B. Fuqua, *Fuqua, A Memoir* (Atlanta: Longstreet, 2001).

20. J. L. Beyer, R. D. Weiner, and M. D. Glenn, *Electroconvulsive Therapy: A Programmed Text*, 2d ed. (Washington, D.C.: American Psychiatric Press, 1998).

21. M. V. Rudorfer, M. E. Henry, and H. A. Sackheim, "Electroconvulsive Therapy," in *Psychiatry*, ed. A. Tasman, J. Kay, and J. A. Lieberman (Philadelphia: W. B. Saunders, 1997), 1535–56.

22. S. Mukherjee, H. A. Sackheim, and D. B. Schnur, "Electroconvulsive Therapy of Acute Manic Episodes: A Review of 50 Years' Experience," *American Journal of Psychiatry* 151 (1994): 169–76.

23. A. Calev, "Neuropsychology and ECT: Past and Future Research Trends," *Psychopharmacology Bulletin* 30 (1994): 461–69.

24. D. J. Kupfer, E. Frank, V. J. Grochocinski, et al., "Demographic and Clinical Characteristics of Individuals in a Bipolar Disorder Case Registry," *Journal of Clinical Psychiatry* 63 (2002): 120–25.

25. A. W. Zobel, T. Nickel, H. E. Kunzel, et al., "Effects of the High-Affinity Corticotropin-Releasing Hormone Receptor 1 Antagonist R121919 in Major Depression: The First 20 Patients Treated," *Journal of Psychiatric Research* 34 (2000): 171–81.

26. J. K. Belanoff, A. J. Rothschild, F. Cassidy, et al., "An Open Label Trial of C-1073 (Mifepristone) for Psychotic Major Depression," *Biological Psychiatry* 52, 5 (2003): 386–92.

27. T. E. Schlaepfer, M. Kosel, and C. B. Nemeroff, "Efficacy of Repetitive Transcranial Magnetic Stimulation (rTMS) in the Treatment of Affective Disorders," *Neuropsychopharmacology* 28, 2 (2003): 201–5.

8. BIPOLAR DISORDER: DIAGNOSIS AND OPTIMAL TREATMENT

1. K. R. Jamison, *Touched with Fire: Manic-Depressive Illness and the Artistic Temperament* (New York: Simon & Schuster, 1993).

2. J. F. Goldberg, T. M. Singer, and J. L. Garno, "Suicidality and Substance Abuse in Affective Disorders," *Journal of Clinical Psychiatry* 62 (Suppl. 25) (2001): 35–43.

3. K. R. Jamison, *An Unquiet Mind: A Memoir of Moods and Madness* (New York: Vintage, 1995).

4. M. C. Blehar, J. R. DePaulo Jr., and E. S. Gershon, "Women with Bipolar Disorder: Findings from the NIMH Genetics Initiative Sample," *Psychopharmacology Bulletin* 34, 3 (1998): 239–43.

5. P. Oswald, D. Souery, and J. Mendlewicz, "Molecular Genetics of Affective Disorders," *International Journal of Neuropsychopharmacology* 6 (2003): 155–69.

6. P. Sklar, S. B. Gabriel, M. G. McInnis, et al., "Family-Based Association Study of 76 Candidate Genes in Bipolar Disorder: BDNF Is a Potential Risk Locus–Brain-Derived Neutrophic Factor," *Molecular Psychiatry* 7, 6 (2002): 579–93.

7. S. S. Ranade, H. Mansour, J. Wood, et al., "Linkage and Association Between Serotonin 2A Receptor Gene Polymorphisms and Bipolar I Disorder," *American Journal of Medical Genetics* 121B, 1 (2003): 28–34.

8. J. C. Soars, "Contributions from Brain Imaging to the Elucidation of Pathophysiology of Bipolar Disorder," *International Journal of Neuropsychopharmacology* 6 (2003): 171–80.

9. P. Linkowski, "Neuroendocrine Profiles in Mood Disorders," *International Journal of Neuropsychopharmacology* 6 (2003): 191–97.

10. S. D. Hollon, R. F. Munoz, D. H. Barlow, et al., "Psychosocial Intervention Development for the Prevention and Treatment of Depression: Promoting Innovation and Increasing Access," *Biological Psychiatry* 52 (2003): 610–30.

11. D. J. Miklowitz, J. A. Richards, E. L. George, et al., "Integrated Family and Individual Therapy for Bipolar Disorder: Results of a Treatment Development Study," *Journal of Clinical Psychiatry* 64, 2 (2003): 182–91.

12. C. L. Bowden, A. M. Brugger, A. C. Swann, et al., "Efficacy of Divalproex Versus Lithium and Placebo in the Treatment of Mania: The Depakote Mania Study Group," *JAMA* 271 (1994): 918–24.

13. R. Hirschfeld, C. L. Bowden, M. J. Gitlin, et al., "Practice Guideline for the Treatment of Patients with Bipolar Disorder (Revision)," *Focus* 1 (2003): 64–110.

14. M. T. Compton and C. B. Nemeroff, "The Treatment of Bipolar Depression," *Journal of Clinical Psychiatry* 61 (Suppl. 9) (2000): 57–67.

15. C. L. Bowden, "Treatment of Bipolar Disorder," in *Textbook of Psychopharmacology*, ed. A. F. Schatzberg and C. B. Nemeroff (Washington, DC: American Psychiatric Press, 1998), 733–45.

16. J. R. Calabrese, C. L. Bowden, G. Sachs, et al., "Placebo-Controlled 18-Month Trial of Lamotrigine and Lithium Maintenance Treatment in Recently Depressed Patients with Bipolar I Disorder," *Journal of Clinical Psychiatry* 64, 9 (2003): 1013–24.

17. Bowden, "Treatment of Bipolar Disorder."

18. M. Tohen, K. N. Chengappa, T. Suppes, et al., "Efficacy of Olanzapine in Combination with Valproate or Lithium in the Treatment of Mania in Patients Partially Non-Responsive to Valproate or Lithium Monotherapy," *Archives of General Psychiatry* 59 (2002): 62–69.

19. M. Tohen, E. Vieta, J. Calabrese, et al., "Efficacy of Olanzapine and Olanzapine-Fluoxetine Combination in the Treatment of Bipolar I Depression," *Archives of General Psychiatry* 60, 11 (2003): 1079–88.

20. J. L. Beyer, R. D. Weiner, and M. D. Glenn, *Electroconvulsive Therapy: A Programmed Text*, 2d ed. (Washington, D.C.: American Psychiatric Press, 1998).

21. N. A. Vaidya, A. R. Mahableshwarkar, and R. Shahid, "Continuation and Maintenance ECT in Treatment-Resistant Bipolar Disorder," *Journal of ECT* 1 (Mar. 19, 2003): 10–16.

22. J. C. Russell, K. G. Rasmussen, M. K. O'Connor, et al., "Long-Term Maintenance ECT: A Retrospective Review of Efficacy and Cognitive Outcome," *Journal of ECT* 1 (Mar. 19, 2003): 4–9.

23. D. J. Kupfer, E. Frank, V. J. Grochocinski, et al., "Demographic and Clinical Characteristics of Individuals in a Bipolar Disorder Case Registry," *Journal of Clinical Psychiatry* 63 (2002): 120–25.

9. REDUCING THE RISK OF SUICIDE

1. A. Alvarez, *The Savage God: A Study of Suicide* (New York: Norton, 1990).

2. Sherwin B. Nuland, *How We Die: Reflections on Life's Final Chapter* (New York: Knopf, 1993).

3. M. Etkind, *Or Not to Be: A Collection of Suicide Notes* (New York: Riverhead, 1997).

4. S. R. Dube, R. F. Anda, V. J. Felitti, et al., "Childhood Abuse, Household Dysfunction, and the Risk of Attempted Suicide Throughout the Life Span," *JAMA* 286 (2001): 3089–96.

5. Ibid.

6. National Center for Health Statistics, *National Vital Statistics Report*, vol. 50, no. 16 (Washington, D.C.: NCHS, Sept. 16, 2002).

7. T. R. Simon, A. C. Swann, K. E. Powell, et al., "Characteristics of Impulsive Suicide Attempts and Attempters," *Suicide and Life-Threatening Behavior* 32 (Suppl.) (2001): 49–59.

8. D. Cremniter, S. Jamain, K. Kollenbach, et al., "CSF 5-HIAA Levels Are Lower in Impulsive as Compared to Nonimpulsive Violent Suicide Attempters and Control Subjects," *Biological Psychiatry* 45, 12 (June 15, 1999): 1572–79.

9. Coalition for Gun Control website: www.guncontrol.ca/Content/Cda-US.htm. Accessed May 22, 2003.

10. H. Hendin, *Suicide in America* (New York: Norton, 1995).

11. C. B. Nemeroff, M. T. Compton, and J. Berger, "The Depressed Suicidal Patient: Assessment and Treatment," *Annals of the New York Academy of Science* 32 (2001): 1–23.

12. S. K. Goldsmith, et al., *Reducing Suicide: A National Imperative* (Washington, D.C.: Institute of Medicine, 2002).

13. W. D. Hall, A. Mant, P. B. Mitchell, et al., "Association Between Antidepressant Prescribing and Suicide in Australia, 1991–2000: Trend Analysis," *British Medical Journal* 326 (2003): 1008–11.

14. R. J. Verkes, R. C. Van der Mast, M. W. Hengeveld, et al., "Reduction by Paroxetine of Suicidal Behavior in Patients with Repeated Suicide Attempts but Not Major Depression," *American Journal of Psychiatry* 155, 4 (1998): 543–47.

15. F. K. Goodwin, B. Fireman, G. E. Simon, et al., "Suicide Risk in Bipolar Disorder During Treatment with Lithium and Divalproex," *JAMA* 290 (2003): 1467–73.

16. American Academy of Child and Adolescent Psychiatry, "Practice Parameter for the Assessment and Treatment of Children and Adolescents with Suicidal Behavior," *Journal of the American Academy of Child and Adolescent Psychiatry* 40, 7 (Suppl.) (July 2001): 24S-51S.

17. Goldsmith et al., *Reducing Suicide*.

10. ANXIETY AND DEPRESSION IN WOMEN

1. R. C. Kessler, P. Berglund, O. Demler, et al., "The Epidemiology of Major Depressive Disorder," *JAMA* 289, 23 (2003): 3095–3105.

2. C. M. Mazure and P. K. Maciejewski, "The Interplay of Stress, Gender, and Cognitive Style in Depressive Onset," *Archives of Women's Mental Health* 6, 1 (2003): 5–8.

3. T. A. Grady-Weliky, "Premenstrual Dysphoric Disorder," *New England Journal of Medicine* 348 (2003): 433–38.

4. K. M. Wyatt, P. W. Dimmock, P. W. Jones, et al., "Efficacy of Vitamin B_6 in the Treatment of Premenstrual Syndrome: Systematic Review," *British Medical Journal* 318 (1999): 1375–81.

5. Grady-Weliky, "Premenstrual Dysphoric Disorder."

6. P. J. Schmidt, L. K. Nieman, M. A. Danaceau, et al., "Differential Behavioral Effects of Gonadal Steroids in Women with and in Those Without Premenstrual Syndrome," *New England Journal of Medicine* 338 (1998): 209–16.

7. M. L. Moline, D. A. Kahn, R. W. Ross, et al., *Postpartum Depression: A Guide for Patients and Families*, Expert Consensus Guideline Series (New York: McGraw-Hill, Mar. 2001).

8. M. Bloch, R. C. Daly, and D. R. Rubinow, "Endocrine Factors in the Etiology of Postpartum Depression," *Comprehensive Psychiatry* 44, 3 (2003): 234–46.

9. This story was posted on the website of the Pacific Post Partum Support Society, www.postpartum.org. Accessed Nov. 21, 2003. Used with permission.

10. K. L. Wisner, B. L. Parry, and C. M. Piontek, "Postpartum Depression," *New England Journal of Medicine* 347 (2002): 194–99.

11. C. D. Chambers, P. O. Anderson, R. G. Thomas, et al., "Weight Gain in Infants Breastfed by Mothers Who Take Fluoxetine," *Pediatrics* 104 (1999): 1120–21.

12. K. Yoshida, B. Smith, M. Craggs, and R. C. Kumar, "Investigation of Pharma-

cokinetics and of Possible Adverse Effects in Infants Exposed to Tricyclic Antidepressants in Breast Milk," *Journal of Affective Disorders* 43 (1997): 225–37.

13. Z. N. Stowe, A. L. Hostetter, M. J. Owens, et al., "The Pharmacokinetics of Sertraline Excretion into Human Breast Milk: Determinants of Infant Serum Concentrations," *Journal of Clinical Psychiatry* 64 (2003): 73–80.

14. G. Stoppe and M. Doren, "Critical Appraisal of Effects of Estrogen Replacement Therapy on Symptoms of Depressed Mood," *Archives of Women's Mental Health* 5, 2 (Oct. 2002): 39–47.

15. D. A. Kahn, M. L. Moline, R. W. Ross, et al., *Depression During the Transition to Menopause: A Guide for Patients and Families,* Expert Consensus Guideline Series (New York: American Menopause Foundation, 2001).

16. H. Joffe, J. E. Hall, C. N. Soares, et al., "Vasomotor Symptoms Are Associated with Depression in Perimenopausal Women Seeking Primary Care," *Menopause* 9, 6 (2002): 392–98.

17. D. S. Charney, R. M. Berman, and H. L. Miller, "Treatment of Depression," in *Textbook of Psychopharmacology,* 2d ed., ed. A. F. Schatzberg and C. B. Nemeroff (Washington, D.C.: American Psychiatric Press, 1998).

18. Writing Group for the Women's Health Initiative Investigators, "Risks and Benefits of Estrogen plus Progestin in Healthy Postmenopausal Women: Principal Results from the Women's Health Initiative Randomized Controlled Trial," *JAMA* 288 (2002): 321–33; C. I. Li, K. E. Malone, P. L. Porter, et al., "Relationship Between Long Durations and Different Regimens of Hormone Therapy and Risk of Breast Cancer," *JAMA* 289 (2003): 3254–63.

19. L. S. Cohen, C. N. Soares, J. R. Poitras, et al., "Short-Term Use of Estradiol for Depression in Perimenopausal and Postmenopausal Women: A Preliminary Report," *American Journal of Psychiatry* 160, 8 (2003): 1519–22.

20. V. Stearns, K. L. Beebe, M. Iyengar, and E. Dube, "Paroxetine Controlled Release in the Treatment of Menopausal Hot Flashes," *JAMA* 289 (2003): 2827–34.

21. J. R. Berman, L. A. Berman, H. Lin, et al., "Effect of Sildenafil on Subjective and Physiologic Parameters of the Female Sexual Response in Women with Sexual Arousal Disorder," *Journal of Sex and Marital Therapy* 27, 5 (2001): 411–20.

11. Anxiety and Depression in Men

1. J. Billingsley, "Bradshaw and Williams Talk About Depression, Anxiety," *Health Scout News,* May 2, 2003.

2. A. M. Moller-Leimkuhler, "Barriers to Help-Seeking by Men: A Review of Sociocultural and Clinical Literature with Particular Reference to Depression," *Journal of Affective Disorders* 71, 1–3 (2002): 1–9.

3. A. M. Minino, E. Arias, K. D. Kochanek, S. L. Murphy, and B. L. Smith,

"Deaths: Final Data for 2000," *National Vital Statistics Reports* 50, 15 (Hyattsville, Md.: National Center for Health Statistics, 2002).

4. S. V. Cochran and F. E. Rabinowitz, *Men and Depression: Clinical and Empirical Perspectives* (San Diego: Academic Press, 2000).

5. W. Pollack, "Mourning, Melancholia, and Masculinity: Recognizing and Treating Depression in Men," in *New Psychotherapy for Men,* ed. W. Pollack and R. Levant (New York: Wiley, 1998), 147–66.

6. J. R. Sibert, E. H. Payne, A. M. Kemp, et al., "The Incidence of Severe Physical Child Abuse in Wales," *Child Abuse and Neglect* 26, 3 (Mar. 2002): 267–76.

7. A. B. Araujo, R. Durante, H. A. Feldman, et al., "The Relationship Between Depressive Symptoms and Male Erectile Dysfunction: Cross-Sectional Results from the Massachusetts Male Aging Study," *Psychosomatic Medicine* 60, 4 (1998): 458–65.

8. P. Cohan and S. G. Korenman, "Erectile Dysfunction," *Journal of Clinical Endocrinology and Metabolism* 86, 6 (2001): 2391–94.

9. R. S. Gregorian, K. A. Golden, A. Bahce, et al., "Antidepressant-Induced Sexual Dysfunction," *Annals of Pharmacotherapy* 36, 10 (2002): 1577–89.

10. L. Barclay, "Sildenafil Effective in Antidepressant-Related Sexual Dysfunction," *JAMA* 289, 1 (2003): 56–64.

11. A. Booth, D. R. Johnson, and D. A. Granger, "Testosterone and Men's Depression: The Role of Social Behavior," *Journal of Health and Social Behavior* 40, 2 (1999): 130–40.

12. H. G. Pope Jr., G. H. Cohane, G. Kanayama, et al., "Testosterone Gel Supplementation for Men with Refractory Depression: A Randomized, Placebo-Controlled Trial," *American Journal of Psychiatry* 160, 1 (2003): 105–11.

13. S. N. Seidman, "Testosterone Deficiency and Mood in Aging Men: Pathogenic and Therapeutic Interactions," *World Journal of Biological Psychiatry* 4, 1 (Jan. 2003): 14–20.

14. W. F. Pirl, G. I. Siegel, M. J. Goode, and M. R. Smith, "Depression in Men Receiving Androgen Deprivation Therapy for Prostate Cancer: A Pilot Study," *Psychooncology* 11, 6 (2002): 518–23.

15. D. J. Selvage and C. Rivier, "Importance of the Paraventricular Nucleus of the Hypothalamus as a Component of a Neural Pathway Between the Brain and the Testes That Modulates Testosterone Secretion Independently of the Pituitary," *Endocrinology* 144, 2 (2003): 594–98.

16. A. J. Kposowa, "Marital Status and Suicide in the National Longitudinal Mortality Study," *Journal of Epidemiology and Community Health* 54, 4 (2000): 254–61.

12. ANXIETY AND DEPRESSION IN CHILDREN AND TEENS

1. The website from which the quotations are drawn is http://teencentral.net.

2. D. Shaffer, P. Fisher, M. K. Dulcan, et al., "The NIMH Diagnostic Interview

Schedule for Children Version 2.3 (DISC-2.3): Description, Acceptability, Prevalence Rates, and Performance in the MECA Study (Methods for the Epidemiology of Child and Adolescent Mental Disorders Study)," *Journal of the American Academy of Child and Adolescent Psychiatry* 35, 7 (1996): 865–77.

3. B. J. Burns, E. J. Costello, A. Angold, et al., "Data Watch: Children's Mental Health Service Use Across Service Sectors," *Health Affairs* 14, 3 (1995): 147–59.

4. D. G. Fassler and L. S. Dumas, *Help me, I'm Sad: Recognizing, Treating, and Preventing Childhood and Adolescent Depression* (New York: Viking, 1997).

5. D. Moreau, "Depression in the Young," *Annals of the New York Academy of Science* 789 (1996): 31–44.

6. F. W. Putnam, "Ten-Year Research Update Review: Child Sexual Abuse," *Journal of the American Academy of Child and Adolescent Psychiatry* 42, 3 (2003): 269–78.

7. Ibid.

8. C. B. Nemeroff, C. M. Heim, M. E. Thase, et al., "Differential Responses to Psychotherapy Versus Pharmacotherapy in the Treatment of Patients with Chronic Forms of Major Depression and Childhood Trauma," *Proceedings of the National Academy of Sciences* 100 (2003): 14293–96.

9. J. F. Rosenbaum, J. Biederman, D. R. Hirshfeld-Becker, J. Kagan, et al., "A Controlled Study of Behavioral Inhibition in Children of Parents with Panic Disorder and Depression," *American Journal of Psychiatry* 157, 12 (Dec. 2000): 2002–10.

10. Anxiety Disorders Association of America, *Conference on Treating Anxiety Disorders in Youth: Current Problems and Future Solutions* (Feb. 2000; monograph).

11. M. B. Stein, M. Fuetsch, N. Muller, et al., "Social Anxiety Disorder and the Risk of Depression: A Prospective Community Study of Adolescents and Young Adults," *Archives of General Psychiatry* 58 (2001): 251–56.

12. J. Kagan and N. Snidman, "Infant Predictors of Inhibited and Uninhibited Profiles," *Psychological Science* 2 (1991): 40–44.

13. J. Biederman, J. F. Rosenbaum, J. Chaloff, and J. Kagan, "Behavioral Inhibition as a Risk Factor for Anxiety Disorders," in *Anxiety Disorders in Children and Adolescents*, ed. J. S. March (New York: Guilford, 1995).

14. D. J. Wiebe, "Homicide and Suicide Risks Associated with Firearms in the Home: A National Case-Control Study," *Annals of Emergency Medicine* 41, 6 (June 2003): 771–82.

15. D. A. Brent and B. Birmaher, "Adolescent Depression," *New England Journal of Medicine* 347 (2002): 667–71.

16. L. Kroll, R. Harrington, D. Jayson, et al., "Pilot Study of Continuation Cognitive-Behavioral Therapy for Major Depression in Adolescent Psychiatric Patients," *Journal of the American Academy of Child and Adolescent Psychiatry* 35 (1996): 1156–61.

17. Brent and Birmaher, "Adolescent Depression."

18. G. J. Emslie, J. H. Heiligenstein, K. D. Wagner, et al., "Fluoxetine for Acute

Treatment of Depression in Children and Adolescents: A Placebo-Controlled, Randomized Clinical Trial," *Journal of the American Academy of Child and Adolescent Psychiatry* 41, 10 (2002): 1205–15.

19. K. D. Wagner, P. Ambrosini, M. Rynn, et al., "Efficacy of Sertraline in the Treatment of Children and Adolescents with Major Depressive Disorder: Two Randomized Controlled Trials," *JAMA* 290, 8 (2003): 1033–41.

20. Public meeting of the Psychopharmacologic Drugs Advisory Committee of the Center for Drug Evaluation and Research, Food and Drug Administration, Washington, D.C., February 2, 2004.

21. Preliminary Report of the Task Force on SSRIs and Suicidal Behavior in Youth. American College of Neuropsychopharmacology, January 21, 2004.

22. Emslie et al., "Fluoxetine for Acute Treatment."

23. P. M. Lewinsohn, D. N. Klein, and J. R. Seely, "Bipolar Disorders in a Community Sample of Older Adolescents: Prevalence, Phenomenology, Comorbidity, and Course," *Journal of the American Academy of Child and Adolescent Psychiatry* 34, 4 (1995): 454–63.

24. B. Geller, B. Zimerman, M. Williams, et al., "Diagnostic Characteristics of 93 Cases of a Prepubertal and Early Adolescent Bipolar Disorder Phenotype by Gender, Puberty, and Comorbid Attention Deficit Hyperactivity Disorder," *Journal of Child and Adolescent Psychopharmacology* 10 (2000): 157–64.

25. E. Leibenluft, D. S. Charney, and D. S. Pine, "Researching the Pathophysiology of Pediatric Bipolar Disorder," *Biological Psychiatry* 53 (2003): 1009–20.

26. B. Geller and J. Luby, "Child and Adolescent Bipolar Disorder: A Review of the Past 10 Years," *Journal of the American Academy of Child and Adolescent Psychiatry* 36, 9 (1997): 1168–76.

27. J. McClellan and J. Werry, "Practice Parameters for the Assessment and Treatment of Adolescents with Bipolar Disorder," *Journal of the American Academy of Child and Adolescent Psychiatry* 36 (Suppl. 10) (1997): 157S–76S.

28. L. K. Vainionpaa, J. Rattya, M. Knip, et al., "Valproate-Induced Hyperandrogenism During Pubertal Maturation in Girls with Epilepsy," *Annals of Neurology* 45, 4 (1999): 444–50.

29. For more detailed information on this subject and specific suggestions for emergency workers, teachers, and other people who work with children, see Helping Children and Adolescents Cope with Violence and Disasters, a website created by the National Institute of Mental Health in the wake of the September 11 attacks; www.nimh.nih.gov/publicat/violence.cfm.

13. ANXIETY AND DEPRESSION IN OLDER ADULTS

1. This story is based on an article by André Picard that appeared in the *Toronto Globe and Mail*, Jan. 9, 2002; used here, in edited form, with permission.

2. G. S. Alexopoulos, S. Borson, B. N. Cuthbert, et al., "Assessment of Late Life Depression," *Biological Psychiatry* 52 (2002): 164–74.

3. G. S. Alexopoulos, "Mood Disorders," in *Comprehensive Textbook of Psychiatry,* 7th ed., vol. 2, ed. B. J. Sadock and V. A. Sadock (Baltimore: Williams and Wilkins, 2000).

4. Y. Conwell, "Suicide in Later Life: A Review and Recommendations for Prevention," *Suicide and Life-Threatening Behavior* 31 (Suppl.) (2001): 32–47.

5. National Mental Health Association, *American Attitudes About Clinical Depression and Its Treatment: Survey Implications for Older Americans* (Alexandria, Va.: NMHA, 1996).

6. C. Salzman, E. Wong, and B. C. Wright, "Drug and ECT Treatment of Depression in the Elderly, 1996–2001: A Literature Review," *Biological Psychiatry* 52 (2002): 265–84.

7. Alexopoulos et al., "Assessment of Late Life Depression."

8. D. S. Geldmacher and P. J. Whitehouse, "Evaluation of Dementia," *New England Journal of Medicine* 335 (1996): 330–36.

9. C. G. Lyketsos and J. Olin, "Depression in Alzheimer's Disease: Overview and Treatment," *Biological Psychiatry* 52 (2002): 243–52.

10. R. C. Green, L. A. Cupples, A. Kurz, et al., "Depression as a Risk Factor for Alzheimer Disease: The MIRAGE Study," *Archives of Neurology* 60, 5 (2003): 753–59.

11. L. Teri, R. G. Logsdon, J. Uomoto, et al., "Behavioral Treatment of Depression in Dementia Patients: A Controlled Clinical Trial," *Journals of Gerontology Series B, Psychological Sciences, and Social Sciences* 52 (1997): 159–66.

12. B. D. Lebowitz, J. L. Pearson, L. S. Schneider, et al., "Diagnosis and Treatment of Depression in Late Life: Consensus Statement Update," *JAMA* 278, 14 (1997): 1186–90.

13. P. A. Arean and B. L. Cook, "Psychotherapy and Combined Psychotherapy/Pharmacotherapy for Late Life Depression," *Biological Psychiatry* 52 (2002): 293–303.

14. Salzman et al., "Drug and ECT Treatment."

APPENDIX II. MAKING SENSE OF HEALTH INFORMATION

1. E. Goodman and J. Capitman, "Depressive Symptoms and Cigarette Smoking Among Teens," *Pediatrics* 106 (2000): 748–55.

2. A. E. Kazdin, "The Meanings and Measurement of Clinical Significance," *Journal of Clinical and Consulting Psychology* 67, 3 (1999): 332–39.

Index

Abilify. *See* aripiprazole
abuse or neglect
  recovery from, 23–24
  recovery of "lost" memories of, 77–78
  as a risk factor for anxiety disorders, 53–54
  as a risk factor for depression, 93, 148, 159–60, 167–68
  and suicide, 138
Academy of Cognitive Therapy, 213
Accutane. *See* isotretinoin
acebutolol, 210
acetylcholine, 110
acne, 183, 210
ACTH. *See* adrenocorticotropic hormone
acupuncture, 201
acyclovir (Zovirax), 211
Adderall. *See* amphetamine
addiction. *See* medications, addiction to; substance abuse
ADHD. *See* attention deficit/hyperactivity disorder
adolescents. *See* children and adolescents
adrenal glands, hormones released by the, 34, 35, 36, 50, 92
adrenaline
  abnormal metabolism of, 67
  amplification by cortisol, 51

physiological effects of, 50
role in fight-or-flight response, 24, 49, 50, 51
role in the mind-body connection, 34
adrenocorticotropic hormone (ACTH), 35, 92
age. *See also* older adults
  differences in symptoms of atypical depression, 89
  and suicide rate, 139
agoraphobia, 66
AIDS, 39, 109
alcohol
  abuse. *See* substance abuse
  and bipolar disorder, 127, 128
  increased risk of depression with, 95
  interaction with antidepressants, 104
  interaction with GABA receptors, 72
Aldomet. *See* methyldopa
Alferon N. *See* interferon
Allerdryl. *See* diphenhydramine hydrochloride
allergic reactions, 209, 210, 211
allostatic load, 26–27
alprazolam (Xanax)
  for anxiety disorder, 179
  case history, 45, 46
  related drugs, 71
  side effects, 94, 210
  tolerance to, 46

half-life of Prozac, 108
hallucinations, 86, 124, 132
Halofed. *See* pseudoephedrine hydro-
    chloride
headache
    with bipolar disorder, 129
    as a risk factor for depression, 39, 40
    as a side effect of medication, 105,
        110, 130
health. *See* mental health; physical
    health
heart disease
    and depression, 31–32, 35, 36–38, 210,
        211
    hormone replacement therapy and
        risk for, 154, 205
    mortality rate, 36
    in older adults, 194
    and traumatic grief, 97
heart palpitations, 110, 199
heart-rate variability, 34, 37
help, finding, 69–71, 212–13
helping others, 25
hepatitis B, 211
herbal medicine, 203
herpes, 211
hippocampus
    ability to grow neurons, 17, 117
    and bipolar disorder, 125
    and memory, 17, 49–50, 62, 93
    size reduction with PTSD, 62
histamine H2-receptor antagonists
    (Axid; Mylanta; Pepcid;
    Tagamet; Zantac), 211
HIV (human immunodeficiency vi-
    rus), 39, 114
HMG-CoA reductase inhibitors, 211
homeopathy, 202
hopelessness
    with dysthymia, 88
    in older adults, 194
    and suicide, 134, 136, 143
hormone replacement therapy (HRT)

depression as side effect of, 154, 155
    for men, 162, 163
    and risk of heart attack, 205
    and risks to women, 154
hormones. *See* growth hormone; sex
    hormones; stress hormones
hospitalization, 117–18, 132, 175
hot flashes, 153, 154, 155
HPA. *See* hypothalamic-pituitary-adre-
    nal axis
HRT. *See* hormone replacement therapy
Hydrocortisone. *See* corticosteroids
hyperforin, 115
hypericin, 115
Hypericum perforatum (Saint John's
    wort), 114–15, 203, 205
hypomania, 121, 122, 123–24
hypothalamic-pituitary-adrenal axis
    (HPA)
    with anxiety and depression, 35
    with behavioral inhibition, 172
    and the menstrual cycle, 148
    overview, 34–36
    with panic disorder, 66
    of suicide victims, 141
hypothalamus
    function of the, 34, 35, 36
    location in the brain, 35
    role in fight-or-flight response, 50–
        51, 92

imipramine (Tofranil), 104, 110, 210
immune system
    and cancer risk with depression, 41
    dampening of, 51
    disorders, 211
    and hormone regulation, 34
impotence. *See* erectile dysfunction
incidence rates
    Alzheimer disease, 196
    anxiety disorders, 47, 192
    depression, 2, 159, 192
    mental illness in children, 166

role in resilience, 26, 199
sodium, low blood level, 131
Sominex. *See* diphenhydramine hydro-
    chloride
spirituality and religion, 25, 140, 157. *See
    also* meaning in life
SRIs. *See* selective reuptake inhibitors
SSRIs. *See* selective reuptake inhibitors
Stanley Medical Research Institute, 216
startle reflex, 64
statins (Lescol; Lipitor; Mevacor;
    Pravachol; Zocor), 211
"statistically significant," 207
statistics used in research, 206–7
steroids, topical, 128
stigma of anxiety and depression
    other people's inability to under-
        stand, 47
    and reluctance to get treatment, 4,
        81, 197
stimulants, use with antidepressants,
    111–12
stomach conditions, 41, 106, 114, 130,
    131, 173
stress. *See also* fight-or-flight response
    childhood, 23–24, 53–55, 93–94
    chronic
        of our culture and times, 2, 92
        as a risk factor for depression, 168
    "inoculation" against, 28, 94
    prenatal, 55
    and resilience, 22, 24, 28
    take time off from, 29
stress hormones
    decreased response during "stress in-
        oculation," 28, 94
    and depression, 92–93
    overview, 92–93
    response to a threat vs. a challenge,
        24
    role in the mind-body connection,
        34–36, 50–52
stroke, 36, 37–38, 194

substance abuse
    with bipolar disorder, 127, 184
    combined with antidepressants, 179
    with dysthymia, 87
    gender differences in, 158
    with generalized anxiety disorder, 64
    importance in treating, 23, 29
    by older adults, 195
    with panic disorder, 65, 128
    by parents, 54, 168, 169
    and PTSD diagnosis, 63
    as self-medication, 58
    and suicide, 134, 136, 138
Sudafed. *See* pseudoephedrine hydro-
    chloride
Sudrin. *See* pseudoephedrine hydro-
    chloride
suicide
    with bipolar disorder, 120
    case history, 133–36
    of a friend, effects on depression, 100
    gender differences, 138, 139, 158, 163
    hospitalization to prevent, 117
    incidence rates, 137, 138, 139, 140, 158,
        175
    "no-suicide pact," 134, 176
    by older adults, 192
    precautions with children or adoles-
        cents, 175
    prevention, 134, 135, 144, 176
    recurrent thoughts of, 86, 106, 173,
        174, 178
    reducing the risk of, 133–44
    and reserpine, 91
    risk factors, 136–42
    screening for tendency toward, with
        TCA, 110
    seen as the logical solution, 83, 84
    and substance abuse, 134, 136, 138
    with traumatic grief, 97
    warning signs, 142–43
    what to do in an emergency, 143–44
suicide notes, 137